the

❸-Plan

your complete **pregnancy**

& postnatal

exercise plan

Lucie Brand

FOR CRIS AND ELISE

Published by Lucie Brand
© 2012 Lucie Brand. All rights reserved.
ISBN 978-0-9572042-0-1

Join the B2MF community!
Web: www.bump2mumfitness.com
Facebook: www.facebook.com/bump2mumfitness
Twitter: bump2mumfit
Blog: bump2mumfitness.blogspot.com

DISCLAIMER

You, the reader, must read and fully understand this release of liability and assumption of risk agreement, fully understand its terms, and agree to it voluntarily without inducement.

'I acknowledge that it is my duty to exercise ordinary care for the protection of others and myself while following the 3-Plan. I assume the risk of physical activity with my own physical condition. I have received advice from my doctor that I am capable of physical exercise such as provided in the 3-Plan, or I will seek such advice, or I will assume the risk of exercising without a doctor's examination. This disclaimer continues to be effective as long as I am following any aspect of the 3-Plan.

I take complete responsibility for my participation and will not hold the 3-Plan responsible for any injuries or loss I may incur as a result of my participation.'

Contents

All about me and the 3-Plan 4

What is the 3-Plan? 6

3-Plan overview 7

Your changing body during pregnancy 12

The benefits of exercising during and after pregnancy 14

All about cardio 16

All about resistance training 18

How do I monitor exercise intensity? 19

Getting to grips with abdominals 20

What can I do if my back aches? 22

Remember to be sensible 23

What about diet? 24

Before and after exercise 28

Chapter 1 The Pregnancy Plan 34

The exercises 36

Section 1 Trimester 1 (weeks 1–12) 37

Section 2 Trimester 2 (weeks 13–26) 50

Section 3 Trimester 3 (weeks 27–40) 63

Running in pregnancy and afterwards 76

Chapter 2 The New Body Plan 78

Section 1 (weeks 0–12 postpartum) 81

Section 1 Part 1 (first six weeks) 81

Section 1 Part 2 (weeks 6–12 postpartum) 82

Section 2 (weeks 13–26 postpartum) 98

Section 3 (weeks 27–40 postpartum) 112

Pelvic floor exercises 125

Common ailments 127

What happens now? 130

Exercise journal template 131

The models have their say 133

Resources 134

Acknowledgements 135

All about me and the 3-Plan

The idea for the 3-Plan came to me when I was in my late twenties and my friends all started having babies. Knowing I was a fitness instructor, they asked me to show them exercises to do during pregnancy that would be safe, which wouldn't harm their babies and would help them get back into shape more easily after the birth.

After doing a little research, it became clear that advice about exercising during and after pregnancy was a bit hit and miss – too complicated in some places, oversimplified in others. Information was hard to relate to and it seemed impossible to find simple, safe, no-nonsense exercises all in one place. The aim of the 3-Plan is to fill this gap.

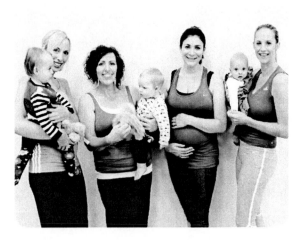

THE CELEBRITY MODEL

These days we are inundated with images of celebrities sporting tiny baby bumps, who are then pictured three or four weeks after giving birth back in their size-zero jeans. Obviously these women have plenty of money and time at their disposal, but this doesn't mean we can't learn from the basic principles of eating right and clever exercising to get a slice of their svelte success.

However, we need to be realistic and patient about our goals. During pregnancy the body goes through a massive transformation and getting back into shape afterwards requires dedication and commitment before and after the birth. The celebs don't wave a magic wand, but they do have a professional dedication to health and fitness.

So I set about designing a flexible exercise programme to follow throughout pregnancy, then after your baby is born – nine months before and nine months after the birth. I used my experience in fitness instruction and personal training with a wide variety of women and studied everything I could about exercising before, during and after pregnancy. I then put together the 3-Plan, which follows all the necessary safety principles.

MY TURN TO TEST THE 3-PLAN

The first draft of the 3-Plan proved brilliant for my friends, who got on really well with it. I then became pregnant myself, so it was my turn to see how effective the 3-Plan really was! It has seen significant changes, based on my friends' feedback and my own experience to result in the book you are reading today. While I was pregnant I worked full time, had a long commute and worked part time as an instructor and trainer, so this was certainly a good road-test of the 3-Plan's flexibility.

I had my beautiful daughter after a short, straightforward labour with no pain relief, which I am convinced was largely due to being fit and healthy. I was amazed at how quickly my body clicked back into shape after the birth. I didn't need nine months, but after following my New Body Plan (the second half of the 3-Plan) my body is in even better shape than before I got pregnant!

THE 3-PLAN WILL HELP YOU, TOO!

So, I've done the hard work for you. The 3-Plan is a unique, easy-to-follow exercise programme; you can fit it in around other commitments and you don't need any expensive equipment. When you get pregnant you are not ill – so embrace this amazing time! Have a go at strengthening your body in preparation for the birth and recovery. You'll need to feel energetic and healthy for life as a mum and there's no need to pile on too many excess pounds, either. You'll feel mentally great, too, as exercise helps fend off the baby blues. You can be a mum with an amazing body – and this really could be the start of a new you! You can be fit and gorgeous for your new family – and, most importantly, for you.

Fitness and me

Since my early twenties I have had a real passion for exercise. After graduating I worked in web design, marketing and communications, always doing lots of exercise in my spare time. When I was 27 I spent over a year training as a fitness instructor and started teaching, quickly building up experience in body conditioning, aerobics, step, spinning and circuits, which made me hungry to pursue a career in the fitness industry.

Since then, I have qualified in nutrition, as a gym instructor and most recently as a personal trainer to help people get the best results from their training.

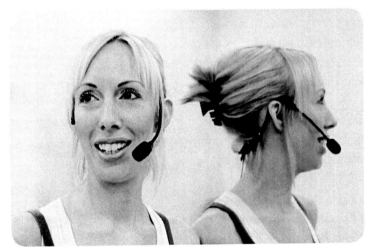

I hope that you will find my book original, fun, motivating and, most of all, effective in helping you to attain your fitness goals.

I specialise in ante- and post-natal fitness, have written and followed the 3-Plan myself and can turn you into a real yummy mummy if you decide to make a commitment to it.

What is the 3-Plan?

The 3-Plan is suitable for anyone and is designed to fit flexibly around your busy life. It produces great results – for your health, fitness and appearance – consisting of a series of resistance exercises designed specifically for your stage of pregnancy or post-natal recovery. It follows the most up-to-date guidance concerning safe exercising for whatever stage you have reached and the exercises change every 12 weeks, helping to keep you motivated!

The idea is that you do the 3-Plan exercises plus moderate cardiovascular activity and a few extras. Why is it called the 3-Plan? The 3-Plan is divided into two main sections: **(1) The Pregnancy Plan** and **(2) The New Body Plan**. Each of these is broken down into three three-month sections. For each section you are given a set of specifically designed resistance exercises. Let's have a quick look at the three main components: resistance training, cardio and extras

1. RESISTANCE TRAINING
Don't be afraid of the term 'resistance' training – it consists of a few simple exercises.

✓ 3 x Leg and bottom exercises
✓ 3 x Upper body exercises
✓ 3 x Ab, back and core exercises

Resistance training will take you between 30 and 40 minutes, three times a week. You also get an extra back up exercise for each body area, just in case you are feeling specially motivated and want to do them all or there is a particular exercise you don't feel confident about doing correctly or which you cannot do due to injury.

For most of the exercises I give you 'easier' and 'harder' options. This way you can really tailor your workout to your fitness level and how you are feeling and progress during each three-month period. If you are feeling great, then do as much as you can, but if you can't manage the standard move go for the easy option – it's far better than doing no exercise at all.

> **WARNING**
>
> If you experience any of the following symptoms you should stop exercising and seek medical advice: vaginal bleeding, being out of breath prior to exercise, dizziness, headache, chest pain, muscle weakness, calf pain or swelling, premature labour, decreased foetal movement, amniotic fluid leakage.
>
> **IMPORTANT**
>
> Make sure you read this section carefully before you begin the exercises.

3-Plan overview

The two halves of the 3-Plan are divided into 3
sections of 3 months (trimesters in pregnancy).
For each section you are given 3 components:
cardio, resistance and extras. For resistance you
have 3 exercises for each body area, plus you get
3 'extras'. The 3-Plan takes a minimum of 3 hours
per week – and that's why it's called the 3-Plan!

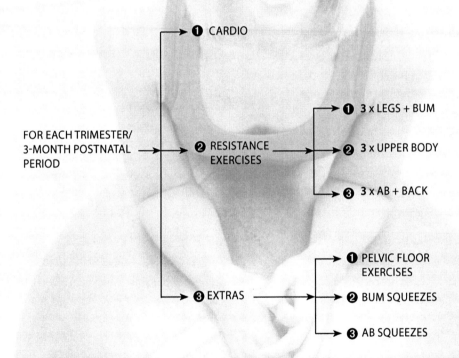

FOR EACH TRIMESTER/
3-MONTH POSTNATAL
PERIOD

❶ CARDIO

❷ RESISTANCE
EXERCISES

❶ 3 x LEGS + BUM

❷ 3 x UPPER BODY

❸ 3 x AB + BACK

❸ EXTRAS

❶ PELVIC FLOOR
EXERCISES

❷ BUM SQUEEZES

❸ AB SQUEEZES

You don't have to do the whole section in one go; do it in chunks! You can do the abs in the morning and the legs and arms later on – whatever suits you best, in whatever order. You can do two sets of each exercise together or mix them up – just try to fit the 3-Plan into your day three times a week.

Compound exercises

Wherever possible the 3-Plan uses 'compound' exercises, which use more than one muscle group (i.e. arms and legs together) and therefore make you work a bit more efficiently and burn more calories. The workout starts with these 'big' exercises and moves on to more isolated ones that target smaller muscles, such as your triceps. There are also some 'super-sets' – two exercises back to back, to really work your muscles hard and tone you up.

2. CARDIO EXERCISES

You need to do at least three cardio workouts per week, which will take you between 20 and 45 minutes. There are easy ways to fit this into your day and the 3-Plan should give you lots of ideas.

What if I'm already super fit?

You may be concerned about not getting enough out of the 3-Plan if you are already a keen exerciser. You will! You can start the 3-Plan straight away and it will help you maintain pre-pregnancy fitness levels.

Some of the effects of pregnancy actually make your body more able to deal with the demands of exercise.

Follow the cardiovascular guidelines, but stick to the higher end of duration and intensity and do the extra resistance exercises if you have time.

PUTTING RESISTANCE & CARDIO TOGETHER

The most straightforward approach is to do your extras every day (or as often as you possibly can) and to work out for about one hour three times a week, each session to include cardio and resistance training. For the very best results you need to try to do at least three further moderate workouts a week for between 20 and 45 minutes; this could perhaps take the form of walking, housework, cycling or gardening (see page 17 for a few more ideas). The 3-Plan is very flexible, though. So just fit in the exercises whenever you can throughout the day, even if it is just in ten-minute chunks whenever you can fit them in.

What if I've never exercised before?

You should wait and start the 3-Plan exercises after your 12-week scan, so go straight in to the Trimester 2 exercises. Follow the cardiovascular guidelines, but stick to the lower end of duration and intensity if you feel more comfortable.

How much time will I need?

You will need to put aside a minimum of three hours per week. You can break this up into small chunks or combine sessions and mix and match cardio activities. The key is to make exercise fun and fit it into your life.

You can't cut corners when it comes to exercise, so if you put in the time and effort and persevere, you will see results. It is also important, particularly while you are following the Pregnancy Plan, to keep momentum going. If you stop halfway through, you may lose some of the benefits.

What do I need to check first?

Anyone can follow the 3-Plan; it doesn't matter if you exercise regularly or if you are completely new to it. The only exception to bear in mind is if you do not have a straightforward 'low-risk' pregnancy. You undertake the 3-Plan at your own risk and it is your responsibility to make sure you are confident that you are not putting yourself or your baby at risk.

From Summary of American College of Obstetricians and Gynecologists (ACOG) 2002.

You should not exercise if you have:

✓ Hemodynamically significant heart disease

✓ Restrictive lung disease

✓ Incompetent cervix/cerclage

✓ Multiple gestation at risk for premature labour

✓ Persistent second- or third-trimester bleeding

✓ Placenta previa after 26 weeks of gestation

✓ Premature labour during the current pregnancy

✓ Ruptured membranes

✓ Preeclampsia/pregnancy-induced hypertension

You should also talk to your Doctor or midwife before undertaking an exercise programme if you have any of the following:

✓ Severe anemia

✓ Unevaluated maternal cardiac arrhythmia

✓ Chronic bronchitis

✓ Poorly controlled type 1 diabetes

✓ Extreme morbid obesity

✓ Extreme underweight (BMI < 12)

✓ History of extremely sedentary lifestyle

✓ Intrauterine growth restriction in current pregnancy

✓ Poorly controlled hypertension

✓ Orthopedic limitations

✓ Poorly controlled seizure disorder

✓ Poorly controlled hyperthyroidism

✓ Heavy smoker

During the 3-Plan you'll never have to do the same exercise twice and the resistance exercises have been put together so that you can progress over the full period.

3. THE EXTRAS

In addition to the main 3-Plan you are also given a variety of pelvic floor, bottom and core strengthening exercises, which you should aim to do as often as possible, whether you are in the supermarket queue, on the bus or while you are watching TV, to really strengthen and prepare these key muscles while you are pregnant and then help

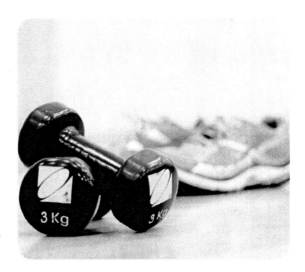

them to get back into shape afterwards. No one will even know you are doing them and these simple moves are super-effective. There are also some moves to ease backache plus some easy stretches later on.

WHAT IS THE PREGNANCY PLAN?

You can follow the nine-month Pregnancy Plan (see pages 34–77) throughout your pregnancy; it is made up of different workouts for each trimester, to suit your body at that stage. The overall aim of this secton of the 3-Plan is to improve your health and fitness levels and to retain and improve muscle tone, keeping you strong, fit, energised and healthy throughout your pregnancy. The Pregnancy Plan is

not an intense training programme and certainly not a diet, but it will help you get back into your pre-pregnancy wardrobe much quicker and make you feel good about yourself, too. It will also help strengthen and prepare your body, for the challenges of pregnancy, childbirth and looking after a new baby.

Lucie says…

"There's plenty of time to get back into shape, so take exercise at your own pace, but try to keep it up."

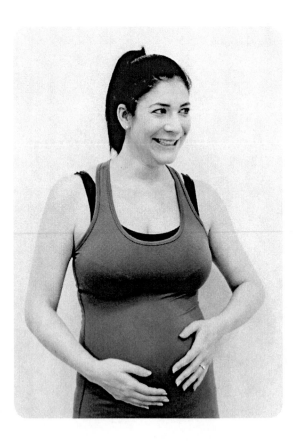

How do I stay motivated?

The 3-Plan will only work for you if you are motivated and positive. So you have to want to make your lifestyle healthier and real results will come about with time and commitment.

To keep yourself going you could put a picture up of yourself when you are at your happiest, to remind you how you want to be, keep a food and exercise diary or reward yourself when you have had a particularly good week – a manicure or pair of shoes rather than a box of éclairs! The overall aim is to develop positive habits that you can stick to for life.

Try to love your figure and feel body-confident. Your positive body image will rub off on your baby and your family and make your world a much happier place. Do what you can to stay fit and healthy, following the 3-Plan, and this should come naturally. Don't strive to be perfect (whatever that is!). Aim to be healthy and happy in your own skin.

What if I have a C-section or a difficult birth?

In the same way that every pregnancy is different, every woman will have a different experience of labour and birth. Some women feel pretty good a few days after giving birth and some take much longer to recover. The main thing to remember about exercising after the birth is to start only when you are ready. A couple of days after – excellent! Six weeks after – also excellent! Start slowly (see the build-up plan on page 81) and listen to your body.

If you have had a C-section or a traumatic birth experience, leaving you with ongoing pain down below, start with walking, ab pull-ins and pelvic floor exercises (which will all help the healing and recovery process) and wait until after you have had your six-week check or feel ready before starting on the full 3-Plan.

WHAT IS THE NEW BODY PLAN?

The nine-month New Body Plan is designed to get rid of all your wobbly pregnancy bits! You can also follow it if you want to tone up and increase your energy and fitness levels (so consider roping in a friend, your partner or your mum for moral support!) This second part of the 3-Plan will help you to lose weight gained during pregnancy and tone up your whole body. Regular exercise will also help relieve stress and give you confidence. The overall aim is to get back to being 'you', so you don't feel as though pregnancy has taken away that inner vixen – she will be back, I promise!

Building up to the New Body Plan, the 3-Plan also gives you a simple six-week exercise schedule to follow directly after you have had your baby. This keeps momentum going and stops your fitness levels falling away, but it allows you as much rest as you need – particularly if you had a difficult delivery – before you embark on the second part of the 3-Plan. You need a little breathing space to bond with your new baby, so remember that these first few weeks of your baby's life are precious – there's loads of time to get back into shape, so take exercise at your own pace.

How will I fit exercise into my day?

There just aren't enough hours in the day are there? Most of us lead very busy lives, leaving very little time for ourselves. However, when you are having a baby or are a new mum it is essential to make time for exercise – for your physical and mental well-being. Even if you can only squeeze in ten minutes a day for a short walk, that's better than nothing. Just focus on the areas of your body you want to work on.

If you are a 'morning person' try getting up earlier than usual, otherwise try a workout while your baby is having a nap, before or after work, or fit in a quick session before dinner.

Let your family and friends know how important exercise is to you and try to build it in to your weekly routine. Once they know, your nearest and dearest may well offer to help out with babysitting or dinner-making to free up some of your precious time.

Accept that every week will probably be different and you may not be able to organise regular exercise slots (a little tricky if you are someone who likes their routines), but build activity and healthy choices into your everyday life and you'll start to see real results.

Your changing body during pregnancy

There are lots of changes going on in your body during pregnancy, but this doesn't mean you can't be active. However, there are a few things to bear in mind.

BE REASSURED

Cool as a cucumber During pregnancy your core temperature rises by approximately 0.6 degrees celsius. Your sweat point lowers, enabling you to dissipate heat from yourself and your baby. This, along with a slightly elevated breathing rate, means that you have a fab inbuilt cooling mechanism and overheating is unlikely.

Go with the flow Cardio exercise will not compromise blood flow to your baby. Provided you are working out at a sensible intensity and not for too long (i.e. over an hour and a half) your body will direct blood to your baby ahead of your working muscles. Stop if muscles feel fatigued.

Added bonus You are still getting all the 'normal' benefits of exercise in addition to the ones related to pregnancy. You'll be boosting your immune system, improving your cardiovascular and muscle fitness and endurance, releasing endorphins and, hopefully, improving your body image.

Put your hands up! Some people say that you shouldn't raise your hands above shoulder height in later pregnancy, in case the umbilical cord gets wrapped around your baby's neck. This is an old wives' tale and you can ignore it. Carry on raising your hands as long as it feels comfortable.

Don't count on it An old school of thought used to say in pregnancy your heart rate during exercise should not go above 140 BPM. There's no right or wrong and every woman is different. A bit of a sweat is OK, but try to keep your effort level moderate – at around 60–70 per cent of your maximum heart rate. Don't measure your heart rate; go by how you feel (see page 19).

BE AWARE

Back in action If you lie on your back (supine) when your bump is big it may put pressure on your vena cava and affect blood flow, making you feel light-headed. This is called 'supine hypotensive syndrome'. Avoid lying on your back for any length of time and try side and seated positions instead.

Full of hot air During pregnancy your need for oxygen increases, meaning your breathing rate rises. Later in pregnancy it also becomes harder to take a big breath as your belly expands. Moderate your workout intensity so you can breathe comfortably.

Huff and puff Progesterone is a hormone that relaxes smooth muscle and makes you more sensitive to CO_2. This may mean your breathing rate increases and you get puffed more quickly. If this happens moderate your intensity.

Working overtime Your resting heart rate (HR) and blood pumped per beat will increase. This means that you should moderate cardio activity as pregnancy progresses. Keep your heart rate up, but make sure you are working at a sensible intensity and not pushing yourself too hard. Also, warm up gradually and steadily decrease intensity at the end of your workout – to bring your heart and breathing rates down gently.

Joint effort The hormone relaxin relaxes your muscles, joints and ligaments, uterus and cervix; this allows your pelvis to open up for the birth. Unfortunately it also affects all your other joints. This doesn't mean you have to put your feet up; just be aware you may be a bit more unsteady and prone to injury during pregnancy, so avoid lots of jumps, twists and tricky footwork.

Vascular underfill When you are first pregnant your body becomes less able to quickly divert your blood to where it is needed. This can make you feel

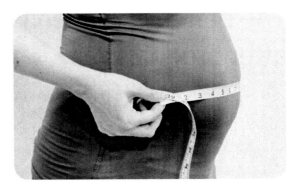

dizzy and faint. If you do, adapt your exercise and avoid quick and frequent transitions (floor to standing etc) and being still for long periods.

What do the experts say about exercise in pregnancy?

In 2002 the American College of Obstetricians and Gynecologists (ACOG) presented the first formal recommendation to include exercise throughout pregnancy, stating, 'in the absence of either medical or obstetric complications, 30 minutes or more of moderate exercise a day on most, if not all, days of the week is recommended for pregnant women' (2002). In support of this the Royal College of Obstetricians and Gynaecologists (RCOG, 2006) suggest that:

✓ All women should be encouraged to participate in aerobic and strength-conditioning exercise as part of a healthy lifestyle during their pregnancy.

✓ Reasonable goals of aerobic conditioning in pregnancy should be to maintain a good fitness level throughout pregnancy without trying to reach peak fitness level or train for athletic competition.

✓ Women should choose activities that will minimise the risk of loss of balance and foetal trauma.

✓ Women should be advised that adverse pregnancy

or neonatal outcomes are not increased for exercising women.

✓ Initiation of pelvic floor exercises in the immediate postpartum period may reduce the risk of future urinary incontinence.

✓ Women should be advised that moderate exercise during lactation does not affect the quantity or composition of breast milk or impact on foetal growth.

The 3-Plan recognises this advice and incorporates it into its exercises programming:

FREQUENCY: 5–7 times a week (encompasses resistance, cardio and daily extras)
INTENSITY: Moderate to hard (see page 19 for how to monitor this)
TIME: 30+ minutes (if possible, otherwise smaller chunks)
TYPE: Recreational not intensive training.

The benefits of exercising during and after pregnancy

In the past many women have been unsure about whether it is safe to exercise during pregnancy or not and have found it hard to get clear advice. These days it is widely accepted that not only is exercise safe during pregnancy, but it has a wealth of benefits and becoming a mum is the perfect opportunity to make regular exercise a part of your life.

The benefits of regular exercise may be...

- ✓ A shorter labour and better endurance, with less likelihood of complications
- ✓ Less likelihood of suffering from nausea and morning sickness
- ✓ Improved core strength and stability
- ✓ A stronger back and reduction in back pain
- ✓ Better posture
- ✓ Stronger pelvic floor muscles
- ✓ Better circulation – less likelihood of suffering from varicose veins, swelling and high blood pressure
- ✓ Stronger bones
- ✓ Less excessive weight gain
- ✓ Better-quality sleep
- ✓ Greater body adaptation to pregnancy

- ✓ More energy and self-confidence – lift your mood and feel great!
- ✓ Stronger muscles (including the ones you use in childbirth)
- ✓ Ability to get in touch with your body, giving you more confidence about labour and recovery
- ✓ Improved cardiovascular fitness and muscle tone
- ✓ Less likelihood of developing gestational diabetes
- ✓ Getting back into shape as a new mum more easily
- ✓ Boosting your immune system
- ✓ Helping to keep baby blues at bay
- ✓ Some 'head space' and time for yourself.

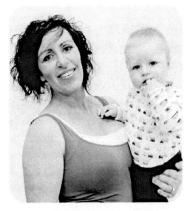

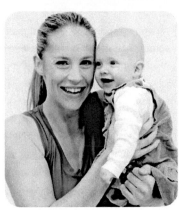

With all of those benefits (see left), why would you not exercise? Well, you may be worried about harming your baby, having a miscarriage, suffering an injury or doing the wrong exercises. The 3-Plan exercises will not harm your baby if you do them properly and will actually offer lots of benefits while he or she is growing inside you. Just do safe and sensible exercise and there really is nothing to worry about. The 3-Plan will have no detrimental effects on your baby while you are pregnant – quite the opposite. In fact, your baby will be less likely to lay down excess fat and will benefit from having a placenta that is larger and more efficient at transporting oxygen, blood and nutrients.

THE EFFECTS OF EXERCISE

After you have had your baby, the effects of the 3-Plan will be positive. Working out with your baby can be a way to bond and spend valuable time together and you will be fitter and have more confidence and energy. Studies show that babies born to exercising mums have equal to, or better, growth and development than those born to non-exercising mums, so it's good news all round.

Lucie says…

"Exercising in pregnancy is a great opportunity for bonding and connecting with your baby."

Will I need any equipment?

You do not need to use any special equipment to do the 3-Plan. Some comfortable clothes and a decent pair of trainers will be all you need to get you started. Some of the exercises require light weights and you can use some 1kg and 3kg hand weights if you wish, but if you don't want to buy them, filled plastic water bottles will provide a good alternative. Weights come in different sizes, so choose the one that is right for you. However, many resistance exercises are effective enough just using your own body weight and a good controlled technique.

If you find the exercises are getting too easy over the three-month period try to increase the weights and opt for the harder moves. In order to work your muscles effectively you need to feel the resistance and it should

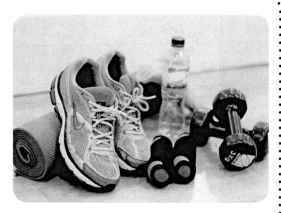

seem as though you can't do any more repetitions once you have completed your set. Don't overdo it in the Pregnancy Plan, though; you can challenge yourself after your baby is born!

All about cardio

The 3-Plan contains cardio elements, which are important for keeping your heart and lungs fit and healthy. There is some flexibility around cardio. You don't have to go to the gym and there are plenty of ways to fit cardio activity into your day.

If you can't fit in three 'proper' cardio sessions try to incorporate cardio activity into your everyday life (see box opposite). If you can get active for at least half an hour between five and seven times a week this will significantly improve your general fitness. Ideally you should do three 'proper' cardio workouts for at least 30 minutes as part of the 3-Plan, for example: jogging, cycling, swimming, cross-training or an exercise class. Two slightly longer sessions (45 minutes+) would be another way to fit cardio in if this suits you better. However, sometimes life gets in the way – don't give yourself a hard time if you are having a 'tired' day. But don't lie to yourself, either; the results you get represent the effort you put in and there are no short cuts.

Chances are that if you just get on and do your workout you'll feel loads better afterwards – glowing and with a sense of pride and achievement. Natural endorphins will give you a fantastic high.

WHAT ELSE CAN I DO?

You don't have to have a home gym or mess up your make-up at the swimming pool to get an effective cardio workout. Your aim is to increase your heart rate and probably get a little bit sweaty. If you are doing the Pregnancy Plan don't be afraid of cardio, it will keep your heart and lungs healthy and strong. You know your limits and fitness levels so

Lucie says…

"Listen to your favourite tunes as you work out, to help motivate yourself."

work at a level that is appropriate for you. A bit of jigging about won't harm your little one. Try the moves listed opposite. I have given you some low- and high-impact alternatives. The low-impact ones are intended for later on in your pregnancy and the initial post-birth period.

Try:
✓ One minute of each twice through the list (opposite)
✓ Two minutes of each once through the list (opposite)
✓ Choose five exercises from the list (opposite) and do each one for three minutes twice.

You get the idea. Mix and match to give you a bit of variety. Stick on your favourite music and get moving. Another option is to draw the curtains and have a boogie in your bedroom!

Everyday cardio

- ✓ Housework
- ✓ Gardening
- ✓ Brisk walking to work or back
- ✓ Using the stairs
- ✓ Leaving the car at home
- ✓ Getting on your bike
- ✓ Playing physical games with your kids
- ✓ Getting off the bus/tube/train a stop early or getting on a stop later
- ✓ Going for a walk at lunchtime or after work
- ✓ Parking a short distance from your destination – building in a walk

Cardio mix and match

- ✓ Half jacks/jumping jacks
- ✓ Skip-on-the-spot/skip-on-the-spot high jumps feet together (rope not essential)
- ✓ Strong march, knees up/jog knees up
- ✓ Alternate heel to bottom/jog heels to bottom
- ✓ Low side-to-side lunge/low side-to-side lunge plus jump to change sides
- ✓ Low hops – four each leg/high jump hops – four each leg
- ✓ Heel digs forward/alternate high kicks forward
- ✓ Twist/twist with jumps and high arms
- ✓ Side-steps/jump side-to-side over centre line
- ✓ Strong wide march/low wide squat jumps
- ✓ Step forward and back/step forward and jump back feet together
- ✓ Lunges backwards/low lunge back plus jump to change sides
- ✓ Jump scissor legs forwards and back (spotty dogs)/ spotty dogs and scissor arms
- ✓ Side steps/side steps with jump, overhead clap
- ✓ Tap to sides/quick pendulum leg swings to sides

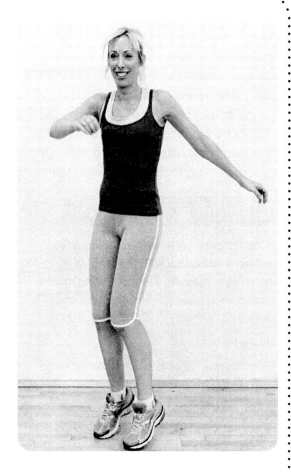

All about resistance training

Resistance training makes your muscles fitter, stronger and more effective and it can be provided by weights, bands or just your body weight. Some people find the term 'resistance training' quite mystifying, even off-putting, but it is key to helping improve muscular fitness, which is extremely important in everyday life, for lifting and carrying things and performing day-to-day tasks.

A good exercise programme, like the 3-Plan, is not limited to cardiovascular training and should incorporate some weight training, too. Once you have seen the results and benefits you'll never be tempted to skip it again. And don't worry about looking like the incredible hulk – you won't bulk up, you'll just increase your strength and maximise the effectiveness of muscle activity. The 3-Plan will tighten and tone your whole body. Remember you should feel a bit hot and sweaty when doing resistance training – you are burning calories and working your heart and lungs, too! Resistance training should be part of your weekly exercise programme if you really want a lean, toned body. You'll be less likely to get injuries too. Start now and you'll see quick results.

The benefits of resistance training

✓ Increases lean muscle, which requires more energy to maintain. It will increase your metabolism, meaning you are burning more calories, even when you are asleep (what could be easier?)

✓ Muscle burns fat

✓ Decreases your risk of developing osteoporosis by increasing bone density

✓ Makes you stronger

✓ Improves your balance, flexibility and core strength

✓ Improves your posture

✓ Makes you feel good and less stressed

✓ Improves your cardiovascular fitness, with all the associated benefits

✓ Shapes and sculpts your body – you'll look more toned and feel great

✓ Increases strength, meaning you have less chance of getting injuries.

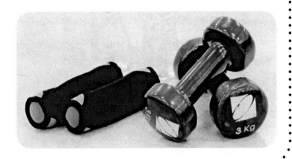

How do I monitor exercise intensity?

When you are exercising it is important to pay attention to exercise intensity. Look at the chart below, relating to your Rate of Perceived Exertion (RPE).

While you are pregnant you should limit your exercise intensity to around 6. This means you can still work hard, feel your heart rate increase and get a bit sweaty, but you shouldn't be pushing your body further than this. When you are following the New Body Plan aim for around 7 or 8, although you won't be able to maintain this for long periods if you are working at a high enough level. Try a little interval training.

Always listen to your body and to work at an intensity that feels right for you. You should be working out effectively, so don't take it too easy, but we don't want any injuries or funny turns, so don't go mad! You'll get to know what your own body can do. Don't forget to use the 'talk test' during pregnancy: you should be able to chat happily while working out.

Rate of Perceived Exertion

- 0 No exercise at all (for example, sitting watching TV)
- 1 Very light
- 2 Fairly light
- 3 Moderate (for example, brisk walking)
- 4 Moderate to hard
- 5 Hard
- 6 Harder (getting a bit sweaty, breathing and heart rate increasing)
- 7 Very hard
- 8 Extremely hard (sweating, heart pumping)
- 9 Even harder (muscles starting to burn a bit)
- 10 Very, very hard (for example, a flat-out super-fast sprint)

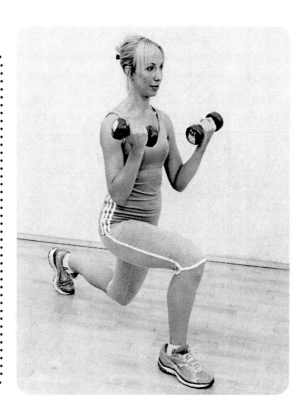

Getting to grips with abdominals

Don't do sit-up-type exercises after Trimester 1 of pregnancy as these put too much stress on weakened surface abdominals. However, it is very important to keep your deep core muscles strong and exercise them regularly to have the best chance of achieving a flat tum again after you have had your baby and minimise the likelihood of getting any pregnancy back pain.

WORK THAT TVA!

That what? The TVA (*transversus abdominis*) is your deepest abdominal muscle and the body's 'internal corset'. You can activate it simply by breathing in deeply and letting your chest expand, then as you exhale, pulling in your tummy all the way around and holding it in for a couple of seconds, then releasing. Gaining control over your TVA and working it as often as possible is key to having a flat tum after you have had your baby. We also call this working your 'core'.

You don't have to do sit-up style exercises to be working your tum. By holding a good posture, keeping a neutral spine and your TVA drawn in throughout your toning exercises you can triple the good work you are doing. You will feel your tummy muscles working, particularly if you are using weights, when you are doing the upper body and leg sections as well as the ab and back sections of the workout. This really engages the core muscles.

DIASTASIS – WHAT IS THAT?

You may have some separation of the abdominal muscles during and after pregnancy (the technical term is 'diastasis', which sounds scarier than it is). This is obvious when you think of how much your

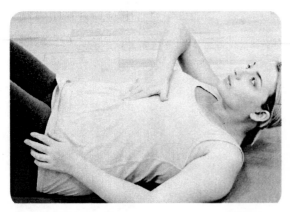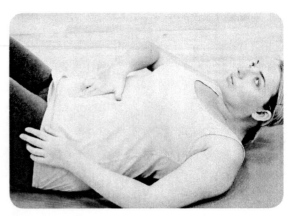

Checking for diastasis

tummy needs to expand to accommodate your little babe. When you have had your baby, you will be able to feel whether you have this separation, or not, with your fingers. Lie on your back, with your feet on the floor, knees bent and head and shoulders lifted. Feel above and below your belly button to see if you can find a gully between your tummy muscles (see pictures below left). By doing the exercises in the 3-Plan, using a good technique, you will be able to gradually close this gap and get a toned, gorgeous tum that you will be proud to show off!

Diastasis separation varies from one person to another, so don't worry if your gap feels quite wide. There are certain exercises that you won't be able to do until the gap has closed to narrower than two finger-widths. Until then you can carry on strengthening your core and helping to close the gap. This is all covered in the New Body Plan (see pages 78–124).

ABDOMINAL SUPPORTS

I found it comfortable to wear an abdominal band to help support my tummy and back while I was exercising, but it is up to you whether you do or don't. My first support was a stretchy band that covered my whole bump for the first six months of pregnancy. Then I switched to an under-the-bump band for the last three. I wore a support most of the time and never experienced any back problems, but do what feels right for you.

WILL THE NEW BODY PLAN HELP MY BABY BULGE?

The abdominals are such important muscles during pregnancy, childbirth and the following months that they warrant a special mention. You might think that because you have had, or are going to have, a baby you can kiss goodbye to that flat-tummy dream. That is simply not the case and you can look even better than you did before.

The Pregnancy Plan will help you to strengthen your deep abdominal muscles, surface abdominal muscles and pelvic floor muscles, ready for childbirth. By working on these before you have your baby you will have a much easier job getting them back into shape afterwards.

The New Body Plan will help you work towards getting rid of your baby bulge. There are three things you need to do to get a flat tummy:

① Get rid of the fat over your tummy by doing cardiovascular exercise.
② Work the deep 'core' muscles to strengthen and tone your tummy and back (these 'partner' muscles need to work together).
③ Tone the surface abdominals.

The New Body Plan covers these three aspects, so stick with it and you will see results. If you have had a C-section you should wait until you have had the go-ahead from your GP and feel ready to begin. (I have used six weeks as a guide and it should be a long enough break for most women. You may choose to start very gently). Also, remember, you may still look pregnant for quite a while after you have had your baby. Again, this is perfectly normal, so don't worry. Everyone's different and it will take some people longer than others to get their figures back; the key is to stick with the 3-Plan and make exercise part of your routine. You are the one in charge of how you change your body.

What can I do if my back aches?

When you are pregnant it is quite common to get an achy lower back. Also, once you have had your baby you will be doing lots of picking up, lifting and bending, which might cause backache, too. So if you get a twinge, give these stretches a try – they should help ease discomfort if you do them regularly.

WARNING
Do not do the exercises in the first column in Trimester 2 or 3.

Lucie says...

"Always listen to your body and to work at a level that feels right for you."

✓ Lie on your back, hugging your knees to your chest.

✓ Lie on your back, with one leg out and the other hugged to your chest.

✓ Lie on your back, with your knees at 90 degrees and feet flat on the floor. Let your knees fall gently to one side, hands to the other. Repeat to the other side.

✓ Lie on your tum with your legs out straight behind you. Prop up on to your elbows and lift your chin to feel a gentle pull on your abs. Be careful not to over-extend.

✓ Lie on your back with your knees bent and feet flat on the floor. Push the small of your back down and into the floor by tightening your lower abdominal muscles.

✓ Lie on your back with your knees bent and feet flat on the floor. Push down through your feet as you slowly lift your bottom off the floor in a bridge.

✓ On all-fours, drop your head, round your spine, hold and release.

✓ Sit in a chair with your feet flat on the floor. Curl your neck, upper back and lower back forwards until your chest is on your thighs and you can touch the ground with your hands.

✓ Stand up straight, arms at your sides and your feet shoulder-width apart. Bend your trunk sideways to the left while sliding your left hand down your thigh and reaching your right arm gently over your head. Repeat to the other side.

✓ Begin in a standing position and exhale as you sweep your arms up sideways and overhead. Tip from the hips and lower into a forward bend, taking your hands towards the floor.

✓ Lower into a squat, with your hands on your thighs and your back arched. Pull your tummy in, round your back up towards the ceiling and drop your head.

✓ On the floor, push back onto your knees, then sit back on your heels as you stretch your arms straight out in front of you, looking down at the floor.

Remember to be sensible

If you are new to exercise, don't try to exercise at the same intensity or level as someone who has been working our regularly for years. You should not take up intensive new activities, such as running during pregnancy, if you have never done them before. The key is to listen to your body and work at your own pace.

You will get to know what feels comfortable and what level is right for you, particularly with cardiovascular exercise (see pages 16–17). If you are feeling unwell or tired, don't beat yourself up about missing a session. The 3-Plan is a long-term programme and acquiring the right habits and making exercise part of your lifestyle is your most important goal.

Most importantly, enjoy the 3-Plan. It is 'you-time' and it should be fun! During pregnancy your whole body will change in ways that you could probably never have imagined, but following the 3-Plan and eating right will mean that these changes won't be permanent and you'll be able to get the 'old' you back. You may embrace your growing bump or miss your flat tummy – either way, the 3-Plan will make you feel the best you can and help you cope with the amazing time of life that is pregnancy, childbirth and motherhood.

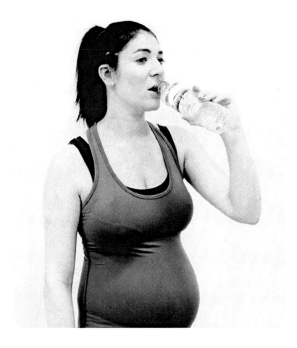

Remember these points

✓ Don't exercise to the point of exhaustion

✓ Wear loose, comfortable clothes and good-quality trainers

✓ Wear a properly fitting sports bra – no flopping about!

✓ Make sure you don't overheat

✓ Stay well hydrated; drink plenty of water

✓ Make sure you do not exercise on an empty stomach or straight after eating

✓ Do not exercise in extreme heat or humidity or run on very rough, hilly ground

✓ Always listen to your body

What about diet?

The 3-Plan is not a diet, but we can't ignore the fact that exercise and nutrition go hand in hand. Some healthy eating advice and calorie guidelines are included here, but bear in mind that this is not meant to be comprehensive.

While you are pregnant, the emphasis should be on eating healthy foods – with the maximum amount of goodness and nutrition to nourish you and your growing baby. You will put on weight and notice it in particular areas, but this is healthy and to be expected.

NICE GUIDANCE

The latest NICE (National Institute for Health and Clinical Excellence) guidance, released in July 2010, says that healthy women who are a normal weight for their height (BMI 18.5–24.9) should gain 11.5–16 kg during pregnancy. Overweight women (BMI 25–29.9) should gain 7–11.5 kg and obese women (BMI greater than 30) should only put on 5–9 kg. So try not to pack on more than this, otherwise you'll still be left with a lot of weight to shift when your baby is born – this isn't healthy for either of you.

Try not to weigh yourself too often. Focus more on how your body looks and feels and remember that lean muscle weighs more than fat.

Lucie says...

"If you've done a good chunk of cardio, make sure you eat something afterwards to help your body recover."

Eating out choices

If you enjoy eating out, don't stop, but try to make healthy choices.

Choose:

✓ Foods that are grilled, boiled or steamed, rather than fried or battered

✓ Options that come with lots of salad or vegetables

✓ Tomato-based sauces rather than creamy ones

✓ Fruit or sorbets for dessert (or share a sweet with a companion)

✓ Drier curries, rather than mild creamy ones

✓ Boiled rice and potatoes rather than fried alternatives

✓ Lean meat and fish with plenty of vegetables

✓ Opt for two courses rather than three

✓ Dressings and sauces 'on the side' rather than on your plate, so that you can decide how much to add

All about calories

If you are a calorie-counter and find this approach helpful, you should try sticking to these approximate calorie guidelines before and after you have your baby.

During pregnancy, in Trimesters 1 and 2
You need 2,000 calories per day, which could be made up of approximately:

✓ Breakfast – 400 calories
✓ Lunch – 400 calories
✓ Dinner – 900 calories
✓ Three healthy snacks of 100 calories each (swap this for a 1 x 300 calorie snack three times a week if you prefer)

You might find you'd rather spread your intake over a few small meals rather than three larger ones; do whatever suits you.

In Trimester 3 and if you are breastfeeding
You need around 2,200–2,300 calories each day:

✓ As above, but add extra calories from a variety of healthy foods

These are only a guide and the main consideration is that your calories should come from the right foods. By following the guidelines on the left you can even have a 300-calorie snack three times a week, which could be a chocolate bar or some other 'naughty' treat!

As a new mum, if you are following the New Body Plan and not breastfeeding:
You will need to cut your calorie intake slightly to start losing weight. I suggest the following as a guideline:

You need 1,600–1,700 calories per day, made up of approximately the following:

✓ Breakfast – 300 calories
✓ Lunch – 300 calories
✓ Dinner – 700–800 calories
✓ Three healthy snacks of 100 calories each (or swap this for a 1 x 300 calorie snack three times a week).

This time, if you can, cut the 'naughty' snacks down to once a week or less. If you are breastfeeding, you can cut down your calories once you have stopped, but remember not to overeat in the meantime.

TO DIET OR NOT TO DIET

Pregnancy is not a time for dieting, but eating whatever you fancy for nine months is not a sensible plan either and losing the extra weight will be much harder.

When you have had your baby you may be breastfeeding (which may help with weight loss), but again, this is not an excuse to eat lots of high-fat, processed foods. This is also not a time to be dieting. You can cut down a bit once breastfeeding is finished. When it comes to losing weight, cut your calorie intake and increase your level of activity – it's as simple as that! Remember

– a regime of chips, cream cakes and no exercise will not help either you or your baby!

Lucie says…

"It's not a good idea to 'eat for two'. You need around 200 calories more per day in Trimester 3 and a bit more if you are exercising, but all your calories should come from healthy foods."

Lucie says...

"Never exercise on an empty stomach. Have a snack about an hour beforehand – a banana, a slice of toast or a cereal bar will give you an energy boost."

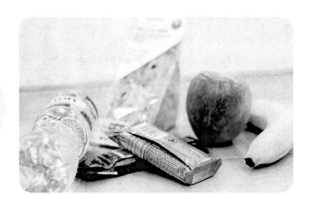

Healthy eating guidelines

Try sticking to the following principles:

✓ Buy lean mince and drain off any excess fat

✓ Buy skimmed or soya milk instead of whole or semi-skimmed milk

✓ Cut any visible fat off meat

✓ Avoid frying. If possible, grill or oven-bake instead. If you do have to fry, use a non-stick pan and a couple of drops of oil or oil spray

✓ Know your Glycaemic Index (GI). Low-GI foods will make you feel fuller for longer, won't give you blood-sugar highs and lows and will keep you fuelled for exercise. The GI value is often stated on food labels

✓ Go for low-fat alternatives (spread, yoghurt, skimmed milk, sauces and mayo)

✓ Have treats in moderation (perhaps just restrict them to three times per week)

✓ Avoid using butter or margarine in sandwiches and on vegetables

✓ Limit your consumption of ready-meals and takeaways

✓ Choose tomato-based sauces and dressings rather than creamy versions

✓ Reduce your intake of cheese

✓ Replace meat with beans and pulses every once in a while

✓ Buy wholewheat pasta, rice and bread, or at least half and half

✓ Use smaller plates to encourage you to reduce your portion sizes if you are trying to lose weight.

✓ Fill half your plate with salad or veggies

✓ Try to increase your fibre intake by eating a high-fibre cereal at least twice a week

✓ Choose fruit and nuts for pudding and snacks instead of sweets and biscuits

✓ Replace saturated fats with 'good' fats from nuts, seeds, oily fish and avocados. Monosaturated fats will help to lower cholesterol in the blood

✓ Use plenty of garlic, spices and seasoning to make your food really tasty and avoid using too much salt

✓ Try to add more fruit and veg to your meals

HEALTHY EATING

Eating healthily is underpinned by a few basic principles. Your diet should be largely based on complex carbohydrates and be made up of a variety of foods including fruit, vegetables, protein and dairy foods, keeping unhealthy processed foods to a minimum. Never is a healthy diet more important than during and after pregnancy.

In this section I have given you some basic advice on how to eat healthily and maximise the nourishment that you and your growing baby are getting from your food. You should avoid gaining excessive weight – it will be much harder to shift later. Your doctor and midwife will be able to tell you throughout pregnancy if you are putting on a healthy amount of weight.

Snacks

Here are some ideas for healthy 100-calorie snacks:

✓ Low-fat yoghurt, mousse or fromage frais

✓ Fruit

✓ Vegetable sticks – celery, carrot, cherry tomatoes and cucumber

✓ Nuts and seeds – but not too many, and not salted nuts

✓ Raisins or other dried fruit

✓ A Weetabix or a small bowl of cereal

✓ Healthy fruit smoothie

✓ Half a bagel or a Ryvita with cottage cheese or a light cream cheese

✓ Cup-a-soup

✓ Low-fat hot chocolate

✓ Crackers or wholemeal toast

✓ Oatcakes or a healthy cereal bar (check the packaging to see whether it really is healthy)

✓ Ricecakes and breadsticks

✓ Ham or tuna with light mayo

✓ A packet of prepared mixed fruit in juice

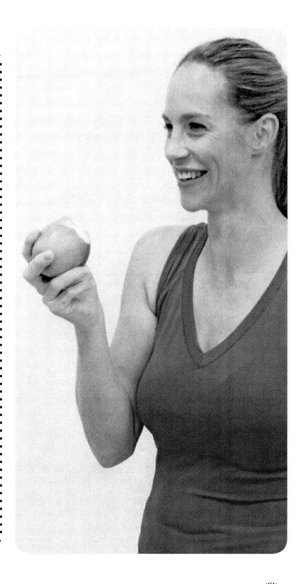

BEFORE AND AFTER EXERCISE

Do I need to do a warm-up?

You need to do a warm-up, but you don't need to spend hours doing it. Time is precious, so just spend a couple of minutes warming up the muscles you will use in your workout. You can also use these moves to cool down, making sure you bring down your heart and breathing rates gradually.

If you don't have time for much of a warm-up, just start off your exercises slowly and build up. Try the exercises below to get your joints mobilised and then to start raising your heart rate a bit:

Ankle rotations and flex and straighten
Stand on one leg, with one foot raised, rotate and point and flex your foot.

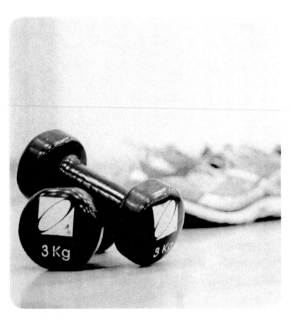

Knee extensions
On one leg, raise one knee, flex your lower leg forwards and back a few times.

Hip rotations both ways
Stand with hands on hips and rotate your hips first in one direction and then in the other.

Twist from waist
Rotate your torso, twisting from side to side with your hands by your temples.

Wrist rotations and flex and straighten
Do this in the same way as for your ankles.

Knee-bends (small squats)
Do a few shallow squats to warm up your knees.

Large parallel arm circles
Have your arms wide and straight and circle them, first forwards and then back.

Large arm-circles cross in front
Move your arms in circular rotations in front of you.

Push arms to sky
Raise your arms and push your hands repeatedly upwards.

Bicep curls
Without weights, flex and straighten the arms.

Shoulder shrugs
Raise your shoulders towards your ears and allow them to drop again.

Shoulder rolls
Rotate your shoulders forwards and back.

Reach arms across/up/down
With one hand on your hip, reach one arm up and bend over to one side. Then repeat on the other side. You can also reach across your body and slide your hand down your thigh as you bend.

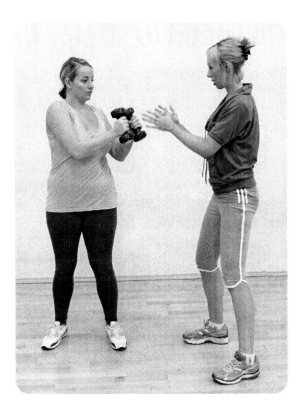

Step touch/step knee lift/step leg curl
Step to the side and back. Add a knee lift or curl with the opposite leg.

Basic step forwards and back
Step forwards and back, taking your feet apart then back together.

March on the spot
As if you are walking but not going anywhere! Lift your knees and swing your arms as you march.

Wide march on the spot
As for March on the spot (above), but feet should be double hip-width apart.

Small side-lunges
Lunge to each side alternately, turning the body slightly. As you lunge, push your opposite arm across your body.

Half jacks
On the same side, take your arm and leg out to the side (step out/punch out). Then repeat on the other side.

Heel digs
Tap your heels forwards alternately. As you dig, bend the other knee and swing your arms forwards.

Small lunges/tap back
Tap your toes back alternately. As you tap back, bend the other knee and curl your arms forwards.

Do I need to stretch?

Try to do a few minutes of stretching after your workout. Just focus on the muscles you have used. For example, you don't need to stretch your arms if you haven't done the arm section of the 3-Plan.

For all the stretches

✓ Keep a neutral spine
✓ Face forwards
✓ Keep your abs pulled in
✓ Keep your shoulders back and relaxed
✓ Keep your joints slightly bent ('soft')
✓ Hold each stretch for eight to ten seconds – to the point of mild discomfort (but not pain!)
✓ Keep your breathing slow and relaxed.

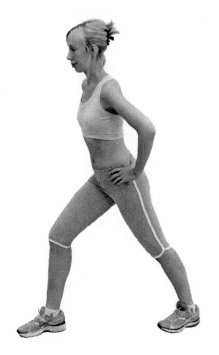

Calf (back of lower leg)
Stand with your feet a hip-width apart. Take a step forwards with one leg, making sure your back heel is down and your front knee is slightly bent. Place your hands on your hips, or wherever is comfortable. Feel the stretch in the lower part of your straight back leg. Then do the same on the other side.

Lucie says…

"Make sure you don't over-stretch as relaxin makes your joints more prone to injury."

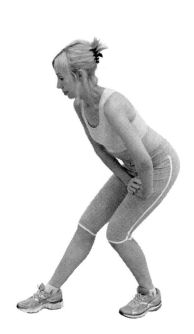

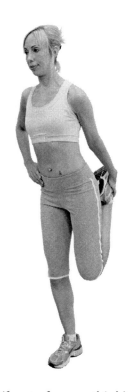

Hamstring (back of upper leg)

Stand with your feet a hip-width apart. Take a step forwards with one leg, making sure your back leg is bent and your front leg is straight, with your toe down. Stick your bottom out and keep your chest lifted. Place your hands on your hips, supporting your leg or wherever feels comfortable. Feel the stretch in the back of your straight front leg. Then do the same on the other side.

Quad (front of upper thigh)

Stand with your feet a hip-width apart, with your knees soft. Lift one heel behind you, up to your bottom. Reach behind to hold on to the front of your foot. Place your other arm on your hip. Feel the stretch in the front of the bent leg. Push your hips forwards to feel the stretch. Then do the same on the other side.

31

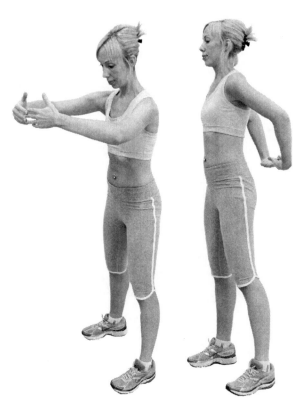

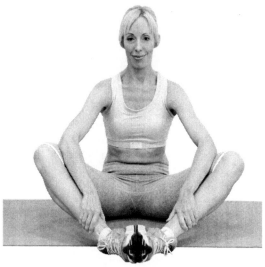

Back and chest

Stand with your feet a hip-width apart. Bring your arms out in front of your body at shoulder height (above left). As you do so separate your shoulder blades and drop your chin to your chest. This will stretch out your upper back. Slowly move your arms wide and behind you, opening up your chest, bringing your shoulder blades together (above right). This will stretch out your chest. Bring your arms back to the starting position.

Inner thighs

Sit upright on the floor. Place the soles of your feet together, as close to your body as is comfortable. Your knees are facing away from your body. Place your elbows on the insides of your knees and put a small amount of pressure on them to feel the stretch in both inner thighs.

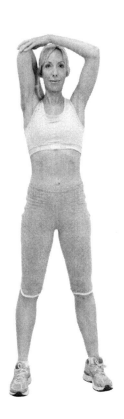

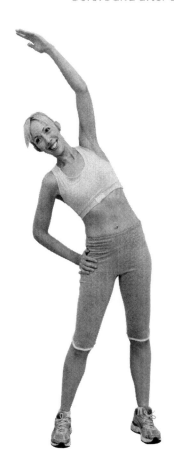

Tricep (back of upper arm)
Stand with your feet a hip-width apart. Lift one arm and bend your elbow, so that your hand goes behind your head, reaching down your back. Use your other hand to push back on your bent arm to increase the stretch. Feel the stretch in the back of your bent arm.

Waist
Lift one arm up to the sky and reach over your head, gently stretching from your waist. Try not to lean forwards or backwards. Then do the same on the other side.

ALTERNATIVES
Other stretches you can try are lying face up on the floor with arms and legs straight to get a full body stretch (but NOT in Trimester 2 or 3), touching your toes to stretch the backs of your legs, twisting from the waist to stretch your side tummy muscles (but not in Trimester 2 or 3) and reaching up, with both arms, to stretch your upper body.

1 The Pregnancy Plan

Congratulations on being pregnant! You are at the start of an amazing journey, which will change you for ever, in both mind and body. At the end of it all you will have a beautiful baby and your life will be transformed. Although this is an incredible time, you may experience a few physical downsides, but I hope that making exercise a part of your life will help you transform negatives into positives and make you the best you can be for your new baby.

You have made the first step and decided to do the 3-Plan. The first part of this book will help you get ready for childbirth and motherhood. If you follow the 3-Plan through pregnancy you will benefit from the positive effects of exercise and be in optimum condition for all the challenges ahead, including getting back into shape as a busy new mum. The Pregnancy Plan is nine months long and is divided into three sections – for Trimesters 1, 2 and 3 of pregnancy. It includes cardio training, resistance training and extras:

❶ CARDIO TRAINING

Try to do 3 x 30–45-minute cardio workouts per week (intensity, type and time depend on pre-pregnancy fitness levels – start with less time if you aren't used to long sessions, gradually building up to 20 minutes or more).

Types of cardio exercise

0–12 weeks (T1) Remember to take it easy if you aren't an experienced exerciser. Perhaps just stick to walking and/or swimming. If you are a seasoned exerciser, there's no reason not to carry on with what you've been doing; just watch your intensity (see RPE, page 19). Avoid rough exercise or contact sports that carry a risk of you being pushed or shoved – use your common sense!

13–26 weeks (T2) This is much the same as Trimester 1. If you are a regular exerciser you can continue with jogging (if you were a runner pre-pregnancy), exercise classes, the gym and most other physical activities. Just be mindful of your growing baby and stop doing anything that makes you feel uncomfortable or unsafe in any way. If you are fairly new to exercise you can also take part in any moderate activity you enjoy – exercise classes, the gym, walking, swimming or anything that makes you a bit sweaty.

27–40 weeks (T3) A bit more caution is required now, but there is no reason to stop doing cardio exercise. Do whatever works for you. You can still jog if you always have and it feels OK; just listen to your body. You may prefer to swap running for brisk walking or alternate walking and jogging (i.e. five minutes of each, alternating). Some gym machines and exercise classes might feel a bit too demanding by now; if so try to find an alternative. Swimming, stationary cycling, cross-training and walking are all excellent. For best results also try to do three further moderate workouts a week for 20–45 minutes; this could be brisk walking, housework, cycling, gardening or anything else that fits into your lifestyle (see pages 16–17).

❷ DAILY EXTRAS

1. Pelvic floor exercises

Try to do three pelvic floor exercises five to seven times a week, or as often as you can (see page 125).

Also do the following extra exercises if you get the chance – at work, on the bus or sitting watching TV – as often as possible. Maybe try making these a part of your daily routine along with your pelvic floor exercises.

2. Bottom-squeezes

To work your bottom, squeeze your bottom muscles as tightly as you can, hold for a couple of seconds and release. Do this 50 times.

3. Ab-squeezes

To work your abs, pull your deep tummy muscles in as tightly as you can (as if you are wearing a really tight corset), hold for a couple of seconds and release. Do this 50 times.

❸ RESISTANCE TRAINING
(3-Plan exercises – different for each trimester)

For each three-month section you have a set of specifically designed resistance exercises suitable for your body in that trimester. This includes:

✓ 3 x leg and bottom exercises
✓ 3 x upper body exercises
✓ 3 x ab, back and core exercises

These will take you 30–40 minutes, three times a week. You also get an extra exercise for each body area for each period. This is just in case you are feeling particularly motivated and want to do them or can be a replacement if there is a certain exercise you don't feel confident about doing correctly or cannot do due to injury.

Remember to add more repetitions or weight or follow the harder alternatives if you feel you are up to working hard or are getting used to the easy options. Follow the basic exercises and easier options if you want a more gentle workout.

If you already do a resistance exercise class, such as Bodypump, you can substitute this for one of your 3-Plan sessions if you prefer, but just make sure you tell your instructor you are expecting.

Two sets of dumbbells are useful (1kg and 3kg).

Lucie says…

"Don't worry about jiggling your baby around; she's tucked up safely in your tum and won't mind! She might even enjoy it!"

THE EXERCISES

I recommend that you have everything you need to hand, so that time doing your exercises is as hassle-free as possible. Get your weights ready, whether they are water bottles, cans of beans or dumbbells. Put on your trainers, crank up your music and you're ready to go! (When exercising on the floor use a mat or rug.)

When you are doing each exercise:

- ✓ Breathe out of the effort of the exercise (the push or pull)
- ✓ Pull your deep core muscles in
- ✓ Use slow and controlled movements; move on counts of two – don't rush!
- ✓ Try to use your full range of movement, flexing and extending your muscles
- ✓ Keep your back and neck neutral throughout
- ✓ Concentrate on the muscle/s you are working and focus on making the movement really effective
- ✓ Don't lock out any of your joints; keep them 'soft' (with a slight bend)
- ✓ Take a short rest between sets
- ✓ If you can do more repetitions or weights, then do more! The numbers given here are just a guide; you need to make sure you can feel your muscles working
- ✓ Don't hold your breath
- ✓ Swap to the easier/harder options if you need to. Try to progress over the 12-weeks period.

Lucie says…

"You don't have to do the whole lot in one go. Just try to fit the 3-Plan into your day, however you can."

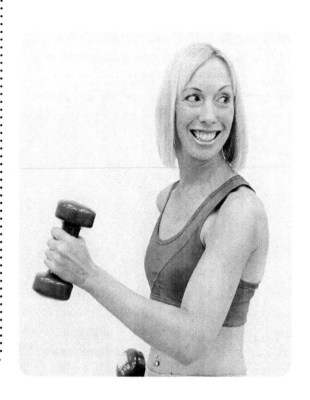

Section 1 Trimester 1 (weeks 1–12)

HOW YOU MIGHT BE FEELING

Although you won't look especially different, you'll be feeling very different! During the first three months of pregnancy the chances are you will feel pretty shattered. In addition to tiredness you may feel sick and be suffering from heartburn, constipation and achy boobs. You might also feel as though you are spending a lot of time on the loo and be quite windy – thhrrrruummp!

Remember; doing some activity may help ease some of these early symptoms, so do your best to stick to the 3-Plan. Exercise can actually give you more energy! You are not limited by your body shape in this first chapter, so I have included some nice big movements to give your new exercise plan a real boost. This is the start of the rest of your life, so try and enjoy it!

Summary

This is an at-a-glance summary of exercises in this section, which you can refer to once you know what you are doing. It's a whole lot easier than flicking through lots of pages each time!

Part 1 Legs and bottom
① Lunge forward and bicep curl (2 x 3kg)
② Squat and rotate (2 x 3kg)
③ Foot pedals (2 x 3kg)
EXTRA Plié-squat and shoulder press (2 x 3kg)

Part 2 Upper body
① Upright row (2 x 3kg)
② Arm-circles
③ Tricep dips
EXTRA Chest-press (2 x 3kg)

Part 3 Abs and back
① Head and shoulder lift
② Abdominal hollowing on all-fours
③ Superman on all-fours
EXTRA Leg cycle

TRIMESTER 1 SAFETY

You can still do more or less what you were doing before you became pregnant, just use your common sense – nothing very high-intensity or dangerous. If you are completely new to exercise, start by walking and swimming, doing the 'extras' and starting the 3-Plan in Trimester 2.

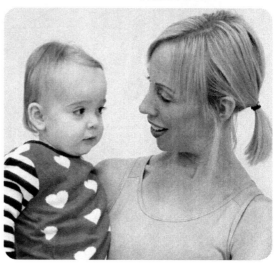

Elise (14 months) and Lucie

PART 1 LEGS AND BOTTOM

1 Lunge forward and bicep curl (2 x 3kg weights)

Your first lower-body exercise is all about getting the basic lunge technique right. This works all your big leg muscles.

① Stand with feet hip-width apart. Hold two weights in your hands, by your sides.

② Step forward with one leg, so that the other back heel comes off the floor and lower your upper body, bending your legs (don't step out too far). Your feet should remain hip-width apart and both knees should be bent at 90 degrees. Keep your upper body upright, with shoulders back and don't lean forwards. Don't allow your front knee to go forwards beyond your toes, as you step forwards.

③ Push up and back to standing and repeat with the other leg.

④ When you are ready, add a bicep curl as you lunge.

Repeat 20 times (alternate legs) and do two sets.

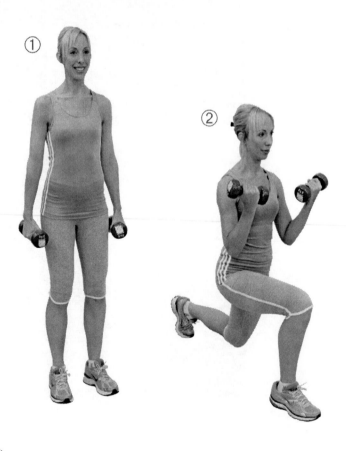

ALTERNATIVES
EASIER   No bicep curl, hands on hips, smaller step forwards
HARDER   Bigger step forwards, deeper lunge, heavier weights, more reps

2 Squat and rotate (2 x 3kg weights)

Your second lower-body exercise is all about getting the basic squat technique right. Again, this will really tone and strengthen your legs.

① Stand with your feet about hip-width apart. Hold a weight in each hand, with your arms bent and the weights just in front of your chest.

② Pull in your abs and keep them tight as you bend your knees and slowly squat, keeping your arms still. Hover, keeping your chin and chest lifted.

③ Push through to lift up and begin straightening your legs. Fully extend your legs until you're back to standing position, but keep your knees soft. As you push up, slowly rotate, twisting from your waist and looking over your shoulder. Always keep your knees in line with your toes and your hands just above your chest. Come back to centre and repeat to the other side.

Repeat 15–20 times (twist to alternate sides) and do two sets.

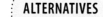

ALTERNATIVES
EASIER Smaller twist, no weights, shallow squat
HARDER Deeper squat, heavier weights, bigger twist – look over your shoulder, add hold in the lowest squat position for ten seconds to finish

①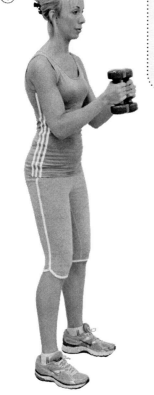

②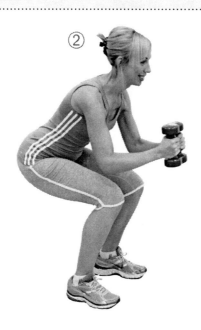

③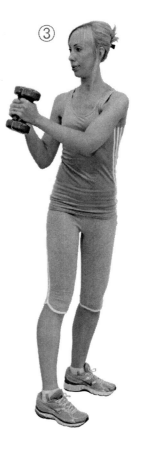

3 Foot pedals (2 x 3kg weights)

Great for toning your calves and bottom and keeping your ankles strong.

① Hold a weight in each hand, with your arms slightly bent and the weights rested on your outer thighs (they stay here throughout). Stand upright, with your shoulders back and abdominals pulled in. Your knees should be slightly bent, feet hip-width apart.

② Gradually raise one heel off the floor, squeezing your calf muscles and your bottom as you do so. Hold for a second and then slowly release.

③ As one heel is coming back towards the floor, start to raise the other heel in a continuous pedalling motion.

Repeat 30–50 times (alternate legs) and do two sets.

②

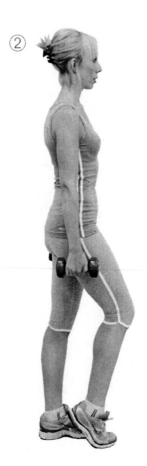

Lucie says...

"You need to really squeeze your bottom as you lift and lower your heels."

ALTERNATIVES
EASIER   No weights, hands on hips
HARDER   Heavier weights, add hammer curls with arms (see page 103)

EXTRA Plié-squat and shoulder press (2 x 3kg weights)

A wider squat will help work those hard-to-reach inner thighs – focus on working them as you squat down.

① Stand with your feet two to three hip-widths apart and your toes pointing outwards, holding two weights.

② Pull in your abs and keep them tight as you bend your knees and slowly squat, keeping your back straight and shoulders back. Your bottom should not push backwards as in the previous squat (see page 39).

③ Hold in the lowest position for a couple of seconds, then fully extend your legs until you're back to the starting position. As you do so, push your arms above your head into a shoulder press (bringing your weights almost together), but keep your knees soft.

Repeat 20 times and do two sets.

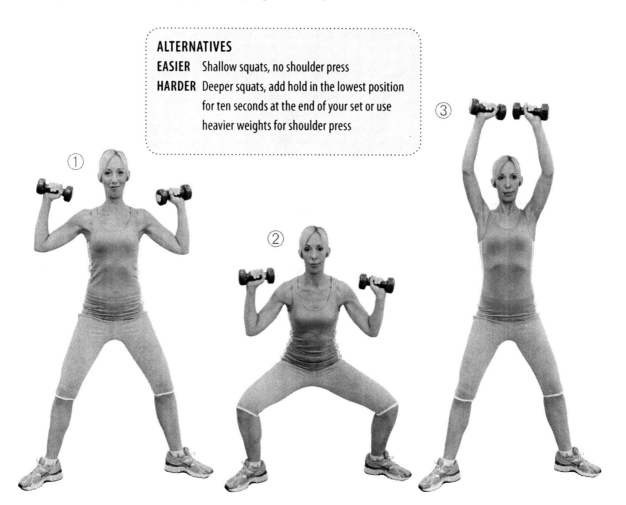

ALTERNATIVES
EASIER   Shallow squats, no shoulder press
HARDER Deeper squats, add hold in the lowest position for ten seconds at the end of your set or use heavier weights for shoulder press

PART 2 UPPER BODY

1 Upright row (2 x 3kg weights)

Great for strengthening your shoulders and arms – these will need to be strong for carrying your baby around.

① Hold a weight in each hand with your arms bent and the weights positioned together, your knuckles facing the ground. Stand up straight with your feet hip-width apart.

② Keeping the weights close to your body, lift them to your chest (midline) level, leading with the elbows.

③ Slowly lower the weights to the starting position. Take care not to round your spine when lifting and keep the action smooth and continuous.

Repeat 15–20 times and do two sets.

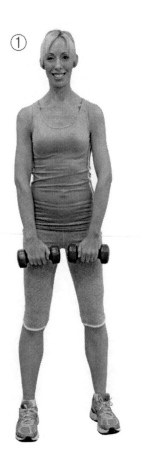

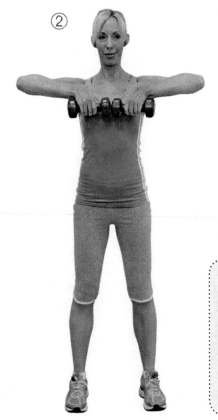

ALTERNATIVES
EASIER Lighter weights
HARDER Heavier weights, then add a set of shoulder pushes at the end (see page 41)

2 Arm-circles

You might feel your arms burning a bit, but keep it going!

① Stand upright, with your shoulders back and abdominals pulled in. Your knees should be slightly bent, your feet hip-width apart. Start with your arms out to the sides, straight, but with a soft elbow, fingers pointed.

② Slowly make circles with each outstretched arm, about 15 cm in diameter.

Do 25–50 forwards, then 25–50 backwards and do two sets.

> **ALTERNATIVES**
> **EASIER** Rest between sets
> **HARDER** Add some light hand weights and keep the circles going for longer!

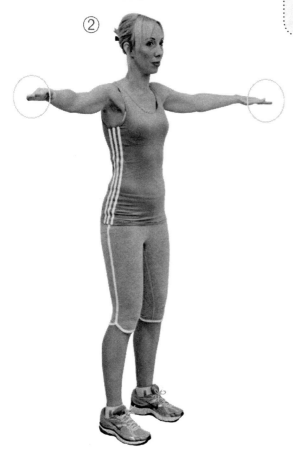

3 Tricep dips

This exercise is fantastic for targeting those pesky bingo wings!

① Sit upright off the edge of a step (or anything stable) with your hands beside you facing forwards (it's very important to have your hands facing towards your toes). Your knees should be bent, with your feet flat on the floor. Lift your bottom up.

② Do a dip by slowly lowering your body to the floor and pushing back up through the triceps, making sure your elbows do not drift out to the sides.

Repeat 15–20 times and do two sets.

ALTERNATIVES
EASIER Feet quite close to your body, shallow dips
HARDER Feet further away or straight legs and deep dips

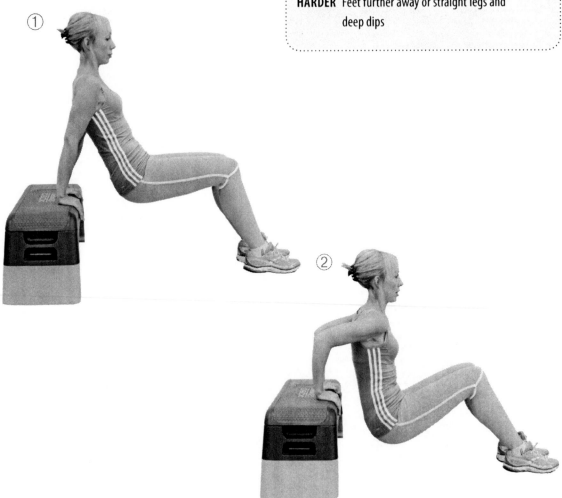

EXTRA Chest-press (2 x 3kg weights)

Keep your chest strong, toned and pert. Remember to get up and down from the floor slowly and carefully. Use an exercise mat or a soft rug/carpet.

(1) Lie on your back with your knees bent and your feet flat on the floor. Hold a weight in each hand with your arms bent at the elbow, resting on the floor and level with the midline of your chest.

(2) Slowly push your arms towards the ceiling, above your chest, until they are almost straight. Then bring them back to the starting position in a controlled way. Remember to keep your tum pulled in, too!

Repeat 15–20 times and do two sets.

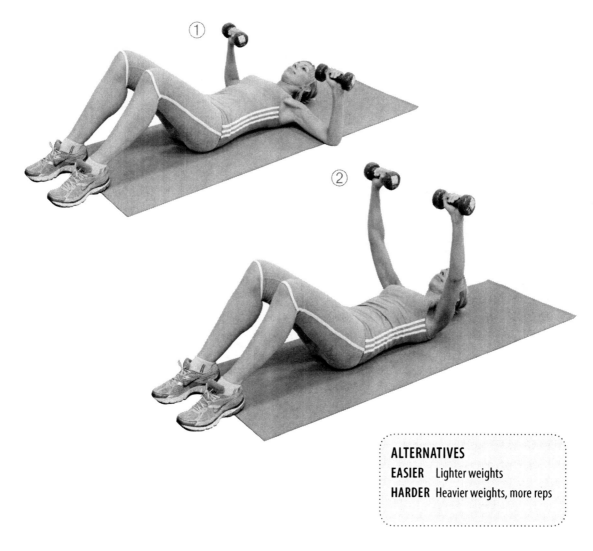

ALTERNATIVES
EASIER Lighter weights
HARDER Heavier weights, more reps

PART 3 ABS AND BACK

1 Head and shoulder lift

Your first ab and back exercise is all about getting the basic technique right to really work your deep core muscles. Be sure to use an exercise mat or a lie on a soft rug/carpet.

① Lie on the floor, with your knees bent and the soles of your feet flat. Breathe in deeply and let your chest expand. Have your hands by your temples.

② Then, as you exhale, draw your belly button in and tilt your pelvis upwards slightly so that your lower back touches the floor or you have a small natural arch.

③ Gradually lift your head and shoulders off the floor towards the ceiling, breathing out as you do so and focusing on pulling your abs in. The rest of your body should be still. There should be a gap between your chin and your chest. Take care not to pull on your neck.

④ Breathe in as you lower again.

Repeat 15–20 times and do two sets.

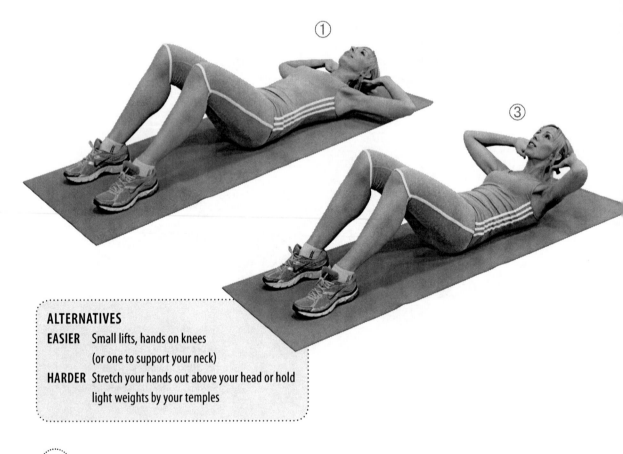

ALTERNATIVES
EASIER Small lifts, hands on knees
(or one to support your neck)
HARDER Stretch your hands out above your head or hold
light weights by your temples

2 Abdominal hollowing on all-fours

This will work your core muscles in a slightly different way.

① On your hands and knees, using a mat, make sure your hands are beneath your shoulders, your knees are hip-width apart and your back and neck are straight.

② Breathe in deeply and let your chest expand. Then as you exhale, draw your belly button in, sucking in your abs all the way around your middle.

③ Hold for a couple of seconds, then release. Make sure you don't arch your back as you pull in.

Repeat 15–20 times and do two sets.

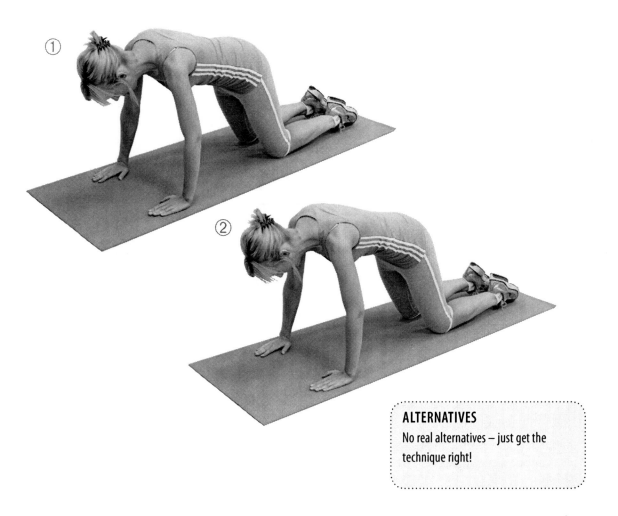

ALTERNATIVES
No real alternatives – just get the technique right!

3 Superman on all-fours

You need good balance for this one; make sure you keep it slow and controlled.

① On your hands and knees, make sure your hands are beneath your shoulders, your knees are hip-width apart and your back and neck are straight.

② When you have pulled your tummy in, lift one leg out straight behind you and the opposite arm straight out in front of you. Keep them lifted for a couple of seconds, making your body as long as possible.

③ Then come back to the starting position. Repeat on the other side.

Repeat 10–15 times (alternate sides) and do two sets.

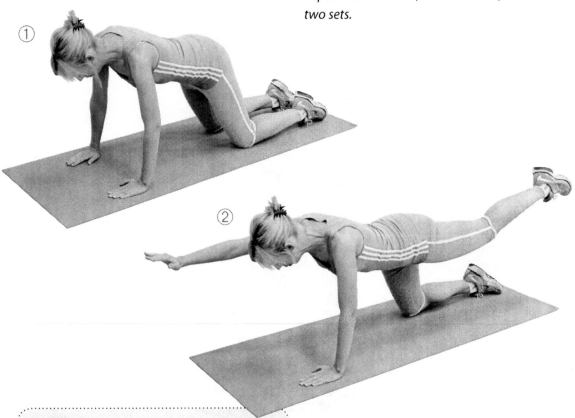

ALTERNATIVES

EASIER   Just lift your arms or legs alternately rather than both together

HARDER Hold the outstretched position for longer (> five seconds) and really reach out

EXTRA Leg cycle

This one is great for targeting your lower abs; a problem area for lots of us!

① Lie on the floor, on a mat, with your knees bent and the soles of your feet flat.

② Breathe in deeply and let your chest expand. Then as you exhale draw your belly button in and tilt your pelvis upwards slightly so that your lower back touches the floor or you have a small natural arch. Have your hands by your sides.

③ With head and shoulders on the floor, lift your legs.

④ Cycle your legs in the biggest circles you can. The rest of your body should remain still. Try to make your leg circles almost touch the floor and bend and fully extend your legs.

Repeat 20–30 times (alternate sides) and do two sets.

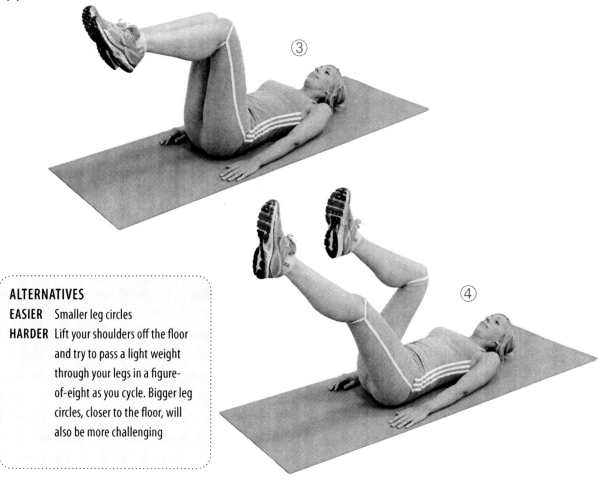

> **ALTERNATIVES**
> **EASIER** Smaller leg circles
> **HARDER** Lift your shoulders off the floor and try to pass a light weight through your legs in a figure-of-eight as you cycle. Bigger leg circles, closer to the floor, will also be more challenging

Section 2 Trimester 2 (weeks 13–26)

HOW YOU MIGHT BE FEELING

You might be feeling any number of things during Trimester 2. You may be full of energy or still suffering from the ravages of morning sickness. Now that you have had your 12-week scan you can be sure that everything is OK (a huge relief!) and confidently get stuck into the 3-Plan – even if you haven't exercised before. Just remember to go at your own pace and listen to your body. You may feel the baby moving or even get some practice contractions in the latter part of this trimester. You may notice a line appearing on your tum; this is called the *linea nigra* and it fades after your baby is born. You might also have more bad wind, piles and varicose veins – oh the glamour! You are going to start looking pregnant sometime soon, if you don't already. You might become a bit light-headed getting up and down, so take your time with transitions. Make the most of this time before your bump gets bigger and remember to try and enjoy every step of your pregnancy. Following the 3-Plan will continue to make you feel good, strong and energised, so keep it up.

Summary

This is an at-a-glance summary of exercises in this section. You can refer to it once you know what you are doing rather than flicking through lots of pages each time.

Part 1 Legs and bottom
① Standing lunge and hammer curls (2 x 1kg)
② Leg lift on all-fours
③ Slow squat
EXTRA Knee-lift and side-lift

Part 2 Upper body
① Standing bicep curl (2 x 3kg)
② Standing tricep kickback (2 x 1kg)
③ Standing narrow bent over row (2 x 3kg)
EXTRA Front-raises (2 x 1kg)

Part 3 Abs and back
① All-fours elbow to knee
② Seated pull-back and ab-hold (2 x 1kg)
③ Standing ab-squeeze
EXTRA Lying leg circles

TRIMESTER 2 SAFETY

Avoid sit-ups, twisting too much, fancy footwork, lying on your back or front for too long and anything unbalanced. Most activities are still fine as long as you start to moderate the frequency and intensity.

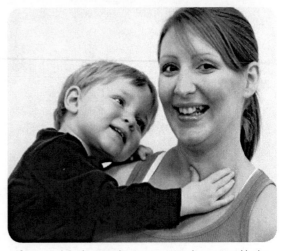

Alfie, 2, and Carly, 34, who is expecting her second baby.

PART 1 LEGS AND BOTTOM

1 Standing lunge and hammer curl (2 x 1kg weights)

Another exercise to work all your big leg muscles – you will also feel this working your supporting leg and bottom.

① Stand with feet hip-width apart, then step forwards on one leg, so you have your legs apart (as if you were going to do a calf stretch – see page 30). Your legs must be wide enough apart so that your back heel is off the ground. You should have your chest lifted, shoulders back and abs in.

② Gradually bend your back knee to 90 degrees, so that it nearly touches the floor, then slowly bring it back up. If you want to make it a bit harder hold a light weight in each hand and hammer curl (see page 103) as you lunge.

Repeat 15–20 times (on each leg) and do two sets

> **ALTERNATIVES**
> **EASIER** Shallow lunge, hands on hips
> **HARDER** Deeper lunge, heavier weights for hammer curls

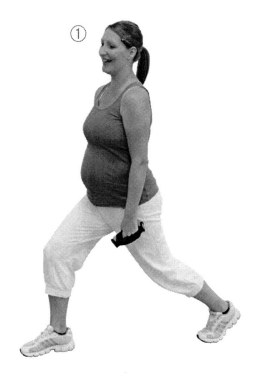

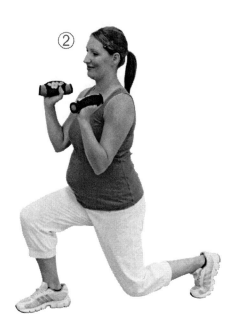

2 Leg lift on all-fours
Work that bottom!

① On all-fours on the floor, rest on your forearms. Extend one leg out behind you in a straight line and lift it about 30 cm off the floor.

② Slowly lift your extended leg, keeping your upper body still, then lower it, keeping it off the floor if you can. This should be a small, controlled movement. Really squeeze your bottom as you lift. Keep your leg high and focus on the upward squeeze.

Repeat 20 times (on each leg) and do two sets.

> **ALTERNATIVES**
> **EASIER** Lower squeeze
> **HARDER** Higher squeeze followed by ten pulses and a ten-second hold at the highest point, really squeezing your bottom

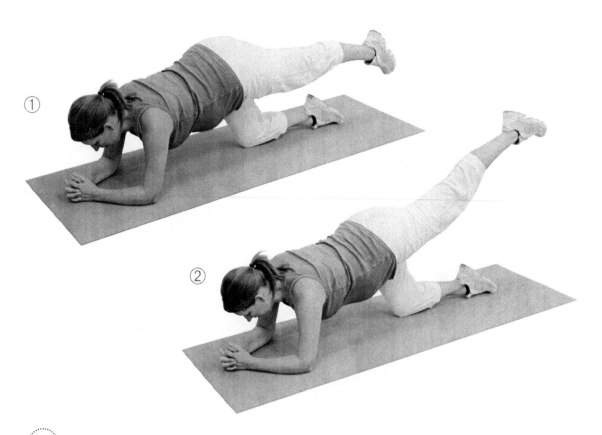

3 Slow squat

By slowing the movement down, you can work the muscles harder; strong legs come in very handy during labour.

① Stand with your feet about a hip-width apart. Pull in your abs and keep them tight as you bend your knees and slowly squat for a count of ten seconds, pushing your arms comfortably forwards.

② Hold briefly in the lowest position, then push through to lift up and begin straightening your legs for a count of ten seconds.

③ Fully extend your legs until you're back to standing position, but keep your knees soft. Always keep your knees in line with your toes.

Repeat ten times and do two sets.

> **ALTERNATIVES**
> **EASIER**   Shallow squats
> **HARDER** Hold light weights on your upper thighs and resist as you squat up and down, do deeper squats, add hold in the lowest position for ten seconds at the end of your set

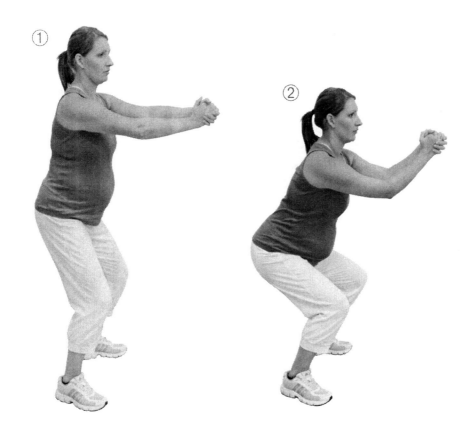

① ②

EXTRA Knee-lift and side-lift

This is a great exercise to mobilise the hip joint (to keep it supple and strong), while working your front and outer thighs.

① Stand with your feet about hip-width apart and your knees slightly bent.

② Keep your shoulders back and look forwards. Pull in your abs and keep them tight as you lift one knee,

③ Then lower your knee without letting your foot touch the floor.

④ Keeping your leg straight, do a side-lift, keeping your raised foot pointing forwards. Go straight into your next knee lift. Do all your reps on one leg, then repeat on the other side.

Repeat 15–20 times (alternate front- and side-lifts) on each leg and do two sets.

ALTERNATIVES

EASIER Just do knee-raises or side-lifts rather than combining the two

HARDER Keep your supporting knee bent and hold some light hand weights. Add ten high side-pulses at the end of your set

---

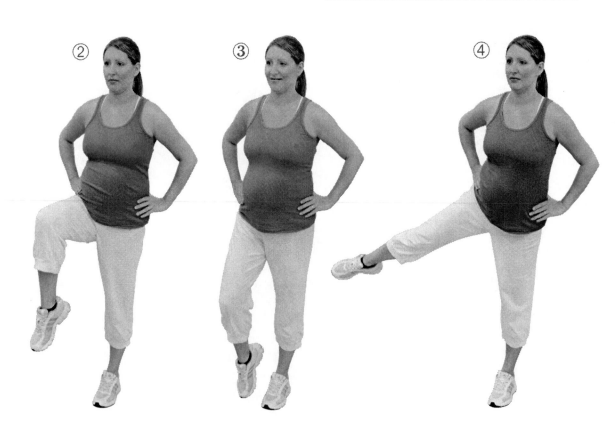

PART 2 UPPER BODY

1 Standing bicep curl (2 x 3kg weights)

You will need strong arms when your baby arrives, so start practising now!

① With your arms straight, hold a weight in each hand. Stand upright, with your shoulders back and abdominals pulled in. Your knees should be slightly bent.

② Slowly curl your arms up as far as you can, then slowly curl back down, with a controlled movement, until your arms are straight and the weights rest on your upper thighs.

Repeat 15–20 times and do two sets.

ALTERNATIVES
EASIER Lighter weights
HARDER Heavier weights, more reps

①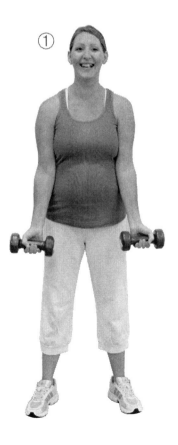

②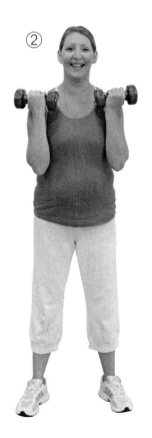

2 Standing tricep kickback (2 x 1kg weights)

Really focus on the tricep muscle as you do this exercise and squeeze the backs of your arms.

① Stand with your feet hip-width apart, then step forwards with one leg so that you have your legs apart (as if you were going to do a calf stretch – see page 30).

② Lean forwards at your waist. Hold a light weight in each hand, with your arms bent at 90 degrees.

③ Slowly extend your arms until they are straight out behind you and squeeze your triceps, pushing your weights upwards. Make sure your arms stay close to your body. Bring your arms back to the starting position.

Repeat 15 to 20 times and do two sets.

ALTERNATIVES
EASIER Don't use any weights
HARDER Use heavier weights and follow your basic set with ten pulses and a ten-second hold at the highest point of your squeeze

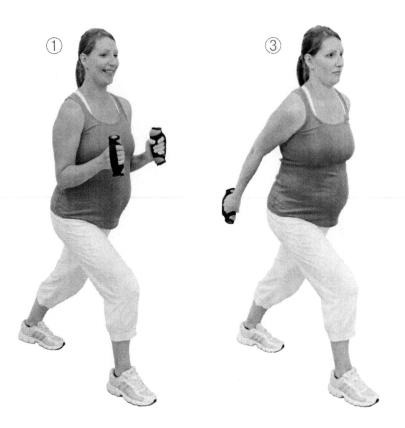

3 Standing narrow, bent over row (2 x 3kg weights)

A nice toned upper back always looks good in strappy tops – really squeeze your shoulder blades together.

(1) Hold a weight in each hand, with your arms straight down by your sides. Stand with your feet hip-width apart, then step forwards with one leg, so you have your legs apart (as if you were going to do a calf stretch – see page 30).

(2) Lean forwards at your waist. Raise your arms in front of you, keeping them straight.

(3) Slowly bend your arms and squeeze your shoulder blades together as you lift your arms and squeeze your upper back. Then slowly return your arms to the starting position.

Repeat 15–20 times and do two sets.

ALTERNATIVES
EASIER Don't use any weights
HARDER Use heavier weights and follow your basic set with a set of wider pulls, with your arms slightly out to your sides

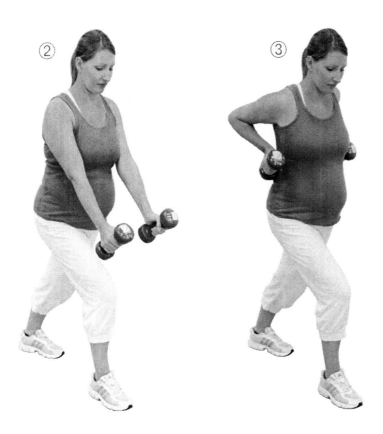

(2)   (3)

EXTRA Front-raises (2 x 1kg weights)

These are quite challenging, so you'll need to work hard to complete your repetitions.

① Hold a light weight in each hand, with your arms straight. Stand upright, with your shoulders back and abdominals pulled in. Your knees should be slightly bent.

② Slowly raise both arms, forwards from your sides to 90 degrees in front of you, keeping your arms straight. Do not raise them above shoulder height. Hold for a couple of seconds, then drop your arms back to your sides, keeping your arms straight.

Repeat 15–20 times and do two sets.

ALTERNATIVES
EASIER Lighter weights
HARDER Heavier weights, more reps

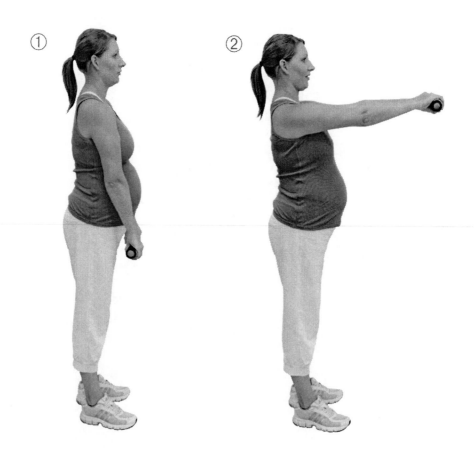

PART 3 ABS AND BACK

1 All-fours elbow to knee

It might be hard to balance to start with. Keep your core strong and your movement slow and controlled.

① On your hands and knees, make sure your hands are under your shoulders, your knees are hip-width apart and your back and neck are straight.

② When you have pulled your tummy in, lift one leg out straight behind you and the opposite arm straight out in front of you (like the Superman, page 48).

③ Slowly bring your arm into your chest and your knee into your tummy without either touching the floor. Hold the crunch for a couple of seconds then return to the starting position.

Repeat 10–15 times (on each side) and do two sets.

ALTERNATIVES
EASIER Stick to a basic Superman (page 48)
HARDER Slow the move right down and try holding a light weight in the moving arm

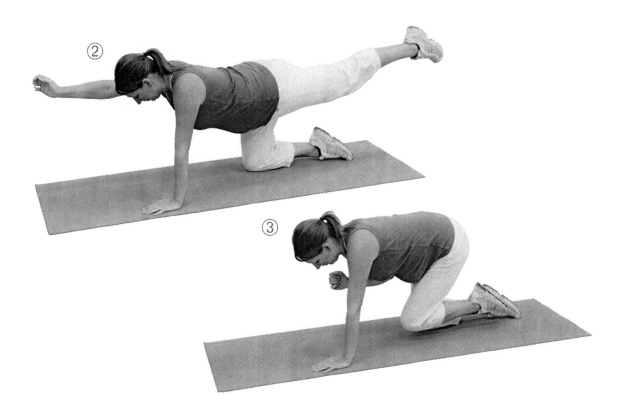

2 Seated pull-back and ab-hold
(2 x 1kg weights)

Work your upper back at the same time as your core – two for the price of one!

① Sit on a chair with your feet on the floor and your back straight. Pull your tummy in and hold it, making sure you can still breathe comfortably.

② Without any weights, hold your arms out in front of you at shoulder height.

③ Slowly pull your arms back, squeezing your shoulder blades together, then return to the starting position. When you have done your repetitions, release your abs.

Repeat 15–20 times and do two sets.

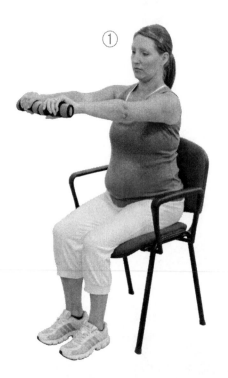

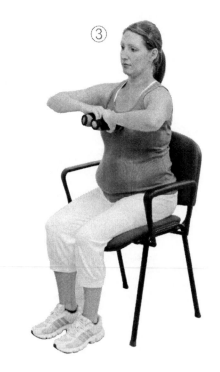

ALTERNATIVES
EASIER Lighter weights
HARDER Heavier weights, more reps

3 Standing ab-squeeze

Do these squeezes as often as possible to make your core super-strong!

① Stand upright with your shoulders back. Breathe in deeply and let your chest expand, then as you exhale draw your belly button in.

② Have your hands by your sides or resting on your belly. The rest of your body should be still. Hold for a couple of seconds, then breathe in as you release.

Repeat 15–20 times and do two sets.

ALTERNATIVES
No real alternatives, just get the technique right!

①

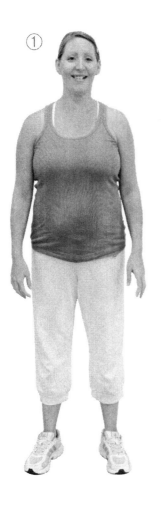

②

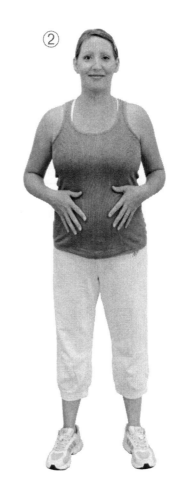

EXTRA Lying leg circles

Although you are mobilising your legs, this is all about core stability. Try and draw the biggest circle you can with your toe!

If you don't want to lie on your back as your bump gets bigger, do this exercise standing up with your tum pulled in and circling each leg one at a time.

① Lie back on the floor with your knees bent and the soles of your feet flat on the floor.

② Breathe in deeply and let your chest expand then as you exhale draw your belly button in and tilt your pelvis upwards slightly so that your lower back touches the floor or you have a small natural arch.

③ Have your hands by your sides. Lift one leg and straighten it so that your toe is pointed.

④ Keeping your leg straight, move it in a big circle slowly outwards, keeping your tummy pulled in. The rest of your body should be still.

Repeat ten times outwards and ten inwards on each leg and do two sets.

> **ALTERNATIVES**
> **EASIER**   Smaller circles, less reps
> **HARDER** Larger circles, more reps, add an ankle weight.

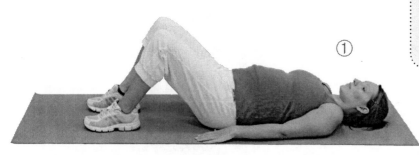

①

Lucie says…

"Don't lie on your back for too long. Sit up between sets. Avoid this exercise if you feel at all faint."

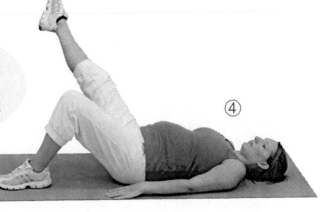

④

Section 3 Trimester 3 (weeks 27–40)

HOW YOU MIGHT BE FEELING

Chances are you'll have a pretty impressive bump by now! You will probably get out of breath and tired at times and may well have some pregnancy-related aches and pains as your body changes to accommodate your growing baby. You may find you are going to the loo a lot and getting practice contractions. Your exercise plan matters more than ever now – keep your muscles, joints and circulation as healthy as possible for both you and your baby.

As crazy as it sounds, doing your 3-Plan exercises and some moderate cardio activity a few times a week will give you more energy than if you do nothing at all! If you miss a session, don't give yourself a hard time; just stick to doing what you can as regularly as possible. Remember, not long to go now until the big day and you need your body to be in tip-top condition – one of the most physically demanding things it will ever go through. All your hard work will make you much more able to deal with the birth. Enjoy these last few weeks! Your baby will soon be here.

Summary

This is an at-a-glance summary of exercises in this section. You can refer to this once you know what you are doing rather than flicking through lots of pages each time!

Part 1 Legs and bottom
① Wide-squat and bicep push forwards (2 x 1kg)
② Calf raise and forward-raise (2 x 1kg)
③ Side-lying leg lift and inner-thigh squeeze
EXTRA Foot-to-sky on all-fours

Part 2 Upper body
① Seated bicep curl and hammer curl (2 x 3kg)
② Standing tricep push-back (2 x 1kg)
③ Standing wall press-up
EXTRA   Seated military press (2 x 3kg)

Part 3 Abs and back
① Standing pelvic tilt
② Seated chest-press and ab-hold (2 x 1kg)
③ Standing squat and ab-hold against wall
EXTRA Standing oblique crunch

TRIMESTER 3 SAFETY

Be mindful of your growing bump and changing body. Don't transition too quickly and keep moves slow and controlled. Perhaps think about choosing low-impact alternatives for your cardio sessions. Don't stop exercising, though, otherwise those hard-earned benefits to you and your baby will be lost.

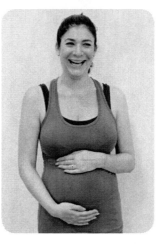

Wendy, aged 31, expecting her first baby.

PART 1 LEGS AND BOTTOM

1. Wide-squat with bicep push-forward (2 x 1kg weights)

Make sure your push-forward is strong to really work those arms!

① Hold a weight in each hand with your arms bent at 90 degrees at your waist. Stand with your feet about two hip-widths apart and toes pointing slightly outwards.

② Pull in your abs and keep them tight as you bend your knees and slowly squat. Keep your chin and chest lifted. Keep your elbows locked into your sides.

③ Push through to lift up and begin straightening your legs. Fully extend your legs until you're back to standing position, but keep your knees soft.

④ As you stand up push your weights forwards, keeping your arms at 90 degrees, until your hands are inline with your head. Squeeze your biceps as you do. Go straight into your next squat.

Repeat 20 times and do two sets.

ALTERNATIVES

EASIER No weights, leave out the push-forward, shallow squat

HARDER Deeper squat, heavier weights, finish with set of push-forwards only

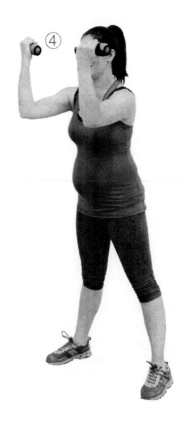

2 Calf-raise and forward-raise (2 x 1kg weights)

You might be experiencing some water retention; these raises are great for mobilising your swollen ankles, in addition to toning your calves and bottom.

① Hold a weight in each hand, with your arms straight and the weights next to your thighs.

② Stand upright, with your shoulders back and abdominals pulled in. Your knees should be slightly bent, feet hip-width apart.

③ Gradually lift both heels off the floor, squeezing your calf muscles and your bottom as you do so. Hold for a second, then slowly release. As you lift your heels, raise both arms up in front of you.

Repeat 20–30 times and do two sets.

ALTERNATIVES
EASIER No weights, hands on hips
HARDER Heavier weights, add a set of quick calf raise pulses at the end of your set

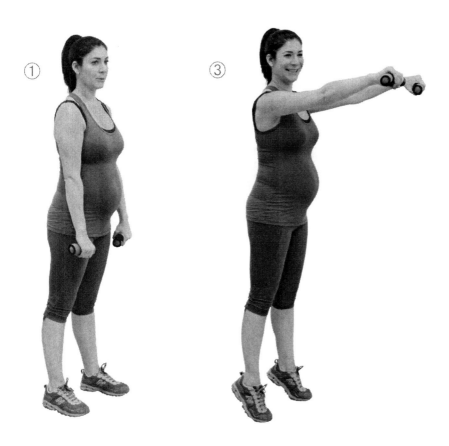

3 Side-lying leg lift and inner-thigh squeeze

Who doesn't want to slimline those problem areas on the insides and outsides of your upper thighs?

Outer thighs

① Lie on your side, with your body in a straight line, one leg bent under you at 90 degrees and your head resting on your hand. Put a pillow under your bump if you like. Make sure your hips are stacked on top of each other.

② Extend your top leg and slowly lift it, keeping your toe pointing forwards and squeezing your outer thigh as you lift.

③ Slowly lower your leg to the starting position. Do all reps without resting your leg.

Inner thighs

④ While still on your side, to work your opposite inner thigh, shift your weight backwards so that you are resting on your elbow and your back leg is bent, with your foot on the floor.

⑤ Extend your front leg out to 45 degrees and slowly lift it, keeping your foot flat and parallel to the floor.

⑥ Squeeze your inner thigh as you lift. Slowly lower the leg to the starting position, but try not to rest it on the floor. Again, do all your reps without resting your leg.

Repeat 15–20 times for each exercise and do two sets. Do both exercises on the other side!

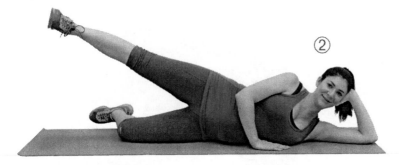

②

ALTERNATIVES

EASIER No weights, hands rested, gentle squeeze

HARDER Rest weights on your outer and inner thighs respectively and add resistance with your hand on both the upward and downward movement

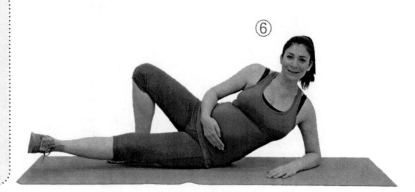

⑥

EXTRA Foot-to-sky on all-fours

Hopefully you will feel a knot in your bottom muscle when you have finished your reps. If not, do some more!

① On all-fours on the floor, have your arms slightly bent, with your hands under your shoulders, looking down at the floor.

② Lift one leg out behind you and push your foot up to the ceiling, squeezing your bottom as you do so.

③ Lower your leg, but keep it fairly high, focusing on the upward squeeze.

Repeat 20 times (on each leg) and do two sets.

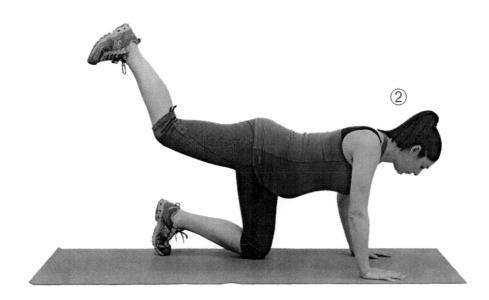

②

ALTERNATIVES

EASIER Gentle squeeze

HARDER Squeeze a light weight behind the knee of the leg you are lifting and hold it there throughout. Follow your reps with ten pulses and a ten-second hold at the highest point

PART 2 UPPER BODY

1 Seated bicep curl and hammer curl (2 x 3kg weights)

Building on a basic bicep curl, adding the hammers will work your arms a bit harder. Don't rest in between the two!

① Sitting down, hold a weight in each hand with your arms straight. Keep your shoulders back and abdominals pulled in.

② To bicep curl, slowly curl your arms up as far as you can, with your palms facing upwards, then slowly curl back down with a controlled movement until your arms are straight.

③ Once you have done your bicep curls, without resting turn your palms to face inwards and curl your arms up in the same way, with the weights pointing up to the sky and complete a set of hammer curls.

Repeat 15–20 times (for each exercise) and do two sets.

ALTERNATIVES
EASIER   Lighter weights
HARDER Heavier weights, more reps

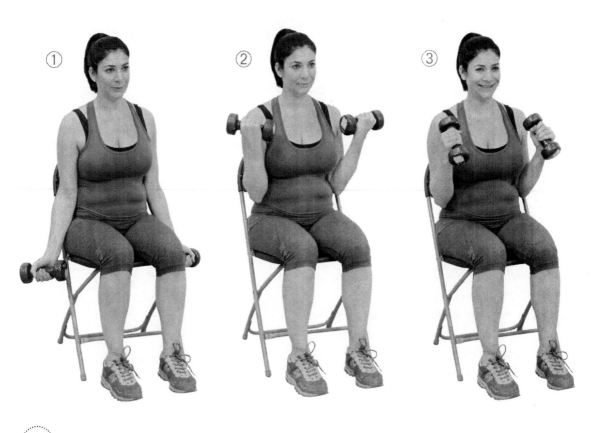

2 Standing tricep push-back
(2 x 1kg weights)

Make sure your upper body doesn't lean forwards; the only movement should be in your arms.

① Stand with your feet hip-width apart, then step forwards with one leg so that you have your legs apart (as if you were going to do a calf stretch – see page 30).

② Hold a light weight in each hand, with your arms straight down by your sides, just slightly pushed back.

③ Slowly lift your arms until they are straight out behind you and squeeze your triceps as you push your palms towards the sky. Make sure your arms stay close to your body. Bring your arms back to the starting position.

Repeat 15–20 times and do two sets.

ALTERNATIVES
EASIER   Lighter weights
HARDER   Use heavier weights and follow your basic set with ten pulses and a ten-second hold at the highest point

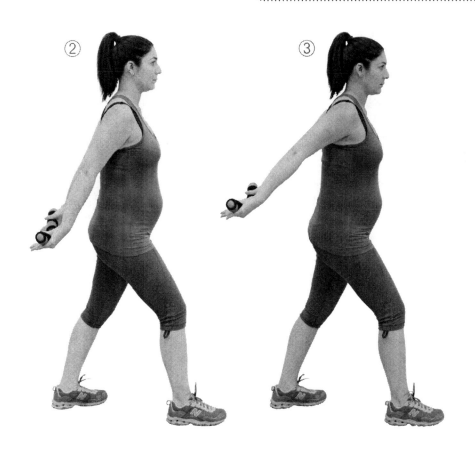

② ③

3 Standing wall press-up

You can make these harder by moving your feet further away from the wall.

① Stand with your feet together, legs straight, abdominals pulled in, shoulders back and head facing forwards.

② Lean forwards and place your hands on the wall at shoulder height. Your heels should be slightly off the floor.

③ Slowly bend your arms and lower your face to the wall, making sure that your whole body moves and your heels roll up off the floor. Push back to the starting position.

Repeat 15–20 times and do two sets.

> **ALTERNATIVES**
> **EASIER** Shallow dip, feet close to wall
> **HARDER** Feet further from wall and add five small low press-ups close to the wall, followed by a five-second hold at the lowest point

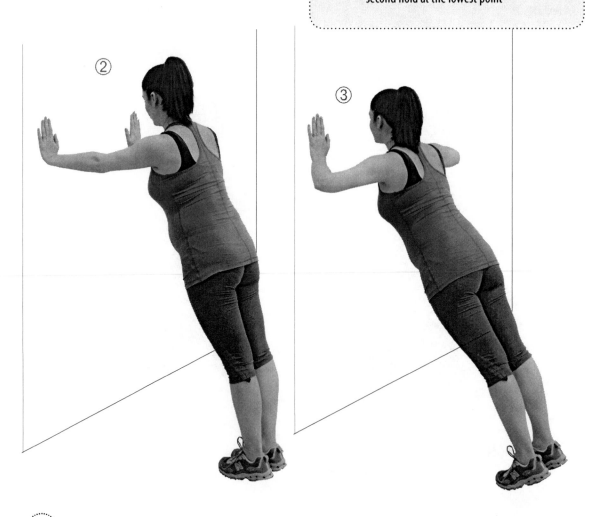

EXTRA Seated military press (2 x3kg weights)

Great for strengthening your shoulders; make sure you pull your core in to keep you strong as you push up.

① Sitting in a chair, hold a weight in each hand with your arms bent and the weights at head height.

② Keep your shoulders back and abdominals pulled in. Slowly push your arms to the sky, but keep them wide; they should not meet.

③ Slowly lower your arms to the starting position, making sure your weights don't drop below head height.

Repeat 15–20 times and do two sets.

> **ALTERNATIVES**
> **EASIER** Lighter weights
> **HARDER** Heavier weights and follow your basic set with a ten-second hold at the highest point

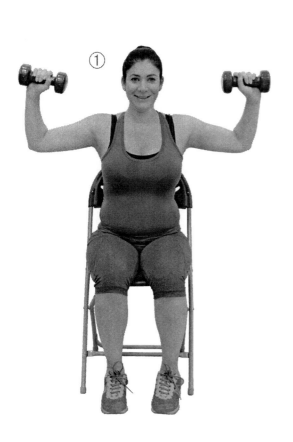

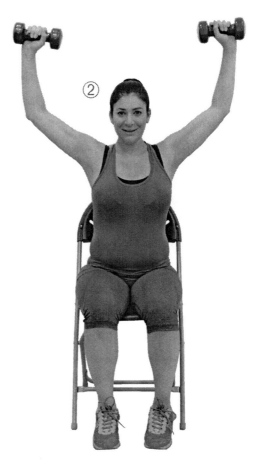

PART 3 ABS AND BACK

1 Standing pelvic tilt

This exercise builds on the basic standing ab-squeeze that we did in Trimester 2 (see page 61). This time you will bring in your pelvis, as well, to really work your core.

① Stand upright, with your shoulders back and your hands on your hips.

② Breathe in deeply and let your chest expand. Then as you exhale draw your belly button in. As you bring your tummy in tilt your pelvis slightly upwards at the same time. The rest of your body should be still.

③ Hold for a couple of seconds, then breathe in as you release.

Repeat 15–20 times and do two sets.

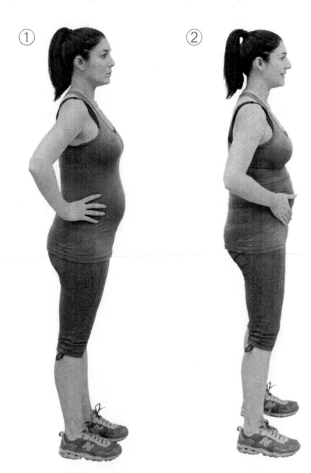

① ②

ALTERNATIVES
No real alternatives, just get the technique right!

2 Seated chest-press and ab-hold (2 x 1kg weights)

This is adding another dimension to the seated ab-squeeze you did in Trimester 2 (see page 60). Tone your upper body at the same time!

① Sit in a chair, with your shoulders back and feet flat on the floor.

② Breathe in deeply and let your chest expand. Then, as you exhale, draw your belly button in so that your lower back touches the back of the chair. The rest of your body should be still. Hold this position, making sure you can breathe comfortably. Hold a light weight in each hand, with your arms bent and the weights at head height. Keep your shoulders back.

③ Slowly bring your arms around to the front, so that your forearms meet and the weights touch. Keep the weights at face height as you do your chest-press.

④ Slowly return your arms to the starting position. Once you have completed your chest-press repetitions release your abs.

Repeat 15–20 times and do two sets.

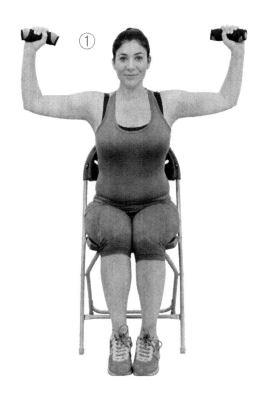

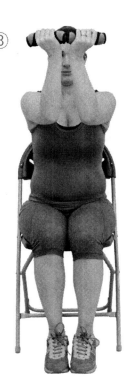

ALTERNATIVES
EASIER Lighter weights
HARDER Heavier weights, more reps

3 Standing squat and ab-hold against a wall

Make sure you have a chair close by to hold on to (not shown), just in case you have trouble getting out of your squat!

① Stand upright, leaning against a wall with your feet hip-width apart. Keep your shoulders back and your chin lifted.

② Slowly squat, sliding your back down the wall. Your legs should be at 90 degrees, if you can manage it. Breathe in deeply and let your chest expand. Then as you exhale draw your belly button in. Have your hands wherever they are comfortable. The rest of your body should be still as you pull your tummy in tight.

③ Hold for five seconds, then breathe in as you release and slide back up. Keep your legs still in the low squat position.

Repeat 15–20 times and do two sets.

ALTERNATIVES
EASIER   Shallow squat, feet close to your body
HARDER   Deeper squat, hold weights on your upper thighs and have your feet slightly further away (but be careful!)

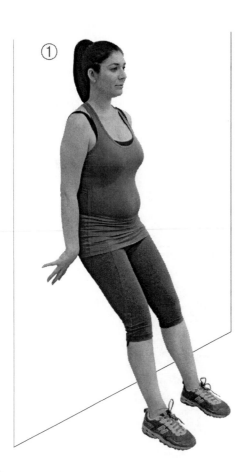

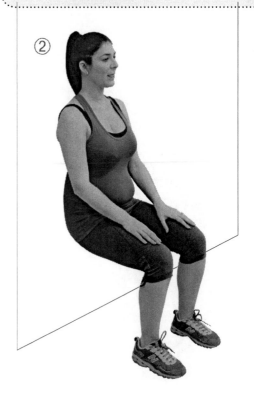

EXTRA Standing oblique crunch

Although you may wonder why you are working your waist while you have an enormous bump, you just have to trust me – that pre-baby waist is still in there!

① Stand upright, with your feet just wider than hip-width apart. Keep your shoulders back and chin lifted. Hold on to the wall with your supporting arm, if you like, and have the other arm bent, with your hand above your head.

② Breathe in deeply and let your chest expand. Then as you exhale draw your belly button in. Make sure you can breathe comfortably.

③ From this position lift your knee out to the side at the same time as you bring your arm down, squeezing the sides of your waist. Hold for a couple of seconds, then release.

Repeat 15–20 times (on each leg) and do two sets.

> **ALTERNATIVES**
> **EASIER**   Just lift your knees
> **HARDER** Hold a light hand weight in the arm that is working

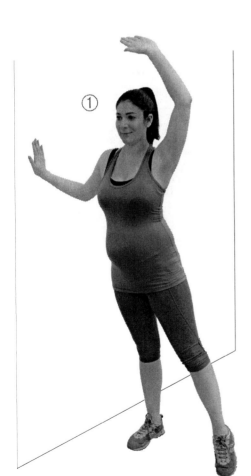

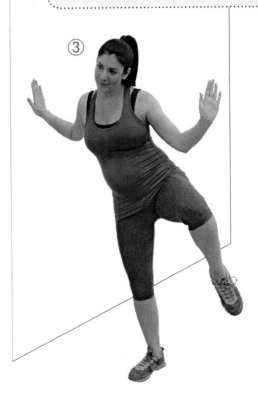

Running in pregnancy and afterwards

One of the most frequent things I hear is that it is not safe to run during pregnancy. However, there is no one-size-fits-all response to this – it largely depends on your pre-pregnancy fitness level and your running experience. If you have never been a runner, do not start during pregnancy.

If you have done a little bit of running I suggest keeping it at a moderate intensity (jogging rather than running) and doing no more than 30 minutes a couple of times a week. If you haven't done any running for at least two months, then do another form of exercise. And if running feels at all uncomfortable then do something else.

If you are an experienced runner then there is no reason why you cannot carry on running during pregnancy. Stick to the safety advice about overheating, clothing, hydration and terrain. Here are some suggested guidelines:

During Trimester 1 carry on as usual, as long as the intensity is not too high (i.e. intervals, sprinting), the duration isn't too long (i.e. longer than 90 minutes) and you are not working harder than you have been used to.

During Trimester 2 start decreasing your intensity and duration once it starts to feel as though it is becoming harder. Remember, you should comfortably be able to maintain a conversation when you are working out. Your body is changing and although you can carry on running (although it should be 'jogging' – not too fast!) you should gradually start to adapt your workouts.

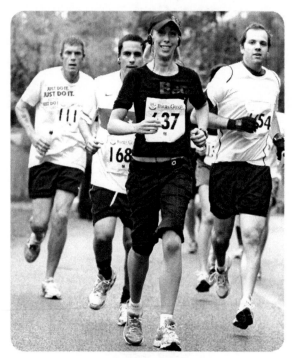

Lucie running the Barnes Green half marathon 14 months after giving birth. She did it in one hour 51!

During Trimester 3 you may be able to carry on jogging if it still feels OK, but make sure you listen to your body and move on to a lower-impact activity if it doesn't feel right. Your bump may make you feel unbalanced or you may experience pelvic aches. Remember that running will put pressure on your pelvic floor as your bump gets bigger. Cross-training, power-walking, cycling and swimming are all great alternatives. If you do continue to jog then work at a comfortable intensity for a sensible duration and maybe build in some walk/jog sessions, alternating for five minutes at a time.

To sum up, if your pregnancy is low risk (see page 9) and you feel fine, don't be frightened to continue running, but remember that it is a high-impact activity and you may feel more comfortable switching to gentler activities later on in your pregnancy. You can always take up running again after the birth (see below). It's up to you – every woman is different.

Ignore anyone who tries to criticise you; we need to change the way people perceive pregnant women – start the revolution! I did my first marathon eight months after giving birth in four hours and 40 minutes.

RUNNING AFTER THE BIRTH

If you want to start running, then you will find advice below to help you build up gradually. Always listen to your body and keep in mind that it has been through a lot. Don't rush.

You can't escape the pelvic floors! Jogging will put pressure on your undercarriage, which will be weakened after childbirth. Even if you had a C-section, your bump would have put pressure on these muscles. If you haven't been doing pelvic floor exercises then start them now if you want to take up running (see page 125). A strong pelvic floor will give you confidence over your wee control while you are running (and the rest of the time, too).

• •

If you are new to running or haven't done any for a while, then start with walking:

① Gradually build up your walks from ten–15 minutes to an hour, walking at a brisk pace. Do this over a period of four–six weeks or until you feel ready to move on.
② After this, build in some walk/jog sessions, alternating between them for five minutes at a time.
③ When you feel comfortable jogging for five minutes, build this up to ten minutes and do this at least five times.
④ Keep adding five-minute blocks on to your runs (doing each duration five times) until you get to where you want to be.

If you are an experienced runner, then you are probably very keen to get back to it!

① For the first four weeks after you have had your baby just follow the first step left.
② When you feel ready, try a gentle 15–20 minute jog. Stop if you experience any discomfort.
③ If this feels OK keep adding five-minute blocks on to your runs (doing each duration five times) until you get to where you want to be. If 15–20 minutes is too much, build up more gradually.

When you are running after having a baby, be sensible. Your body and pelvis, in particular, has been through an ordeal so you need to let your body adapt to each step of your running programme before you move on.

2 The New Body Plan

You've done it – you're a mum! Well done you! Giving birth is amazing, life-changing, scary, exciting and surreal – all at the same time! You are now starting out on a brand-new life with your new family. It really is up to you how quickly you want to get back to exercising again. The main priority is to enjoy spending time with your new baby in the early days; after all, you can never get these moments back again.

The 3-Plan is very flexible and designed to fit around your life, and after labour and the birth process it is completely adaptable to whatever birth experience you have had and how you are feeling. You may want to start working your abs and pelvic floor again within a couple of days of giving birth – which you can if you like. But you may equally want to wait six weeks before you do anything at all. Whatever your decision, start the New Body Plan when you are ready. The main thing is that you *do* do it and that you stick with it.

If you had a C-section, you can do the Weeks 1 and 2 build-up plan exercises, but you should wait until you get the all-clear from your GP (this usually happens around six weeks after the birth) before you do any more.

If you are breastfeeding that is fantastic. You can still exercise – just wear a good supportive bra, with breast pads if necessary. Keep any cardio exercise to moderate-high intensity and wait until you have finished breastfeeding to really push yourself hard with very high-intensity cardio sessions.

If you had any stitches down below these can be sore for a while, so take it easy until everything feels OK and you've been given the all-clear by your GP. Your pelvic floor exercises will help you heal, though, so do these if you can.

The New Body Plan is nine months long and is divided into three sections, each three months long. The plan includes cardio, training, resistance training and extras:

❶ CARDIO TRAINING

Try to do 3 x 30–45-minute cardio workouts per week (intensity, type and time depends on pre-pregnancy fitness levels – start with less if you are a beginner and build up to 20 minutes).

0–3 weeks postpartum Walking only. See the six-week build-up plan (see page 81).

3–40 weeks postpartum It is very individual as to what cardio exercise you want to do after you have your baby – and when you do it. If you feel comfortable reintroducing cardio exercise after three weeks, then start again slowly. If you prefer to wait until your six-week check-up then wait. The main thing is that from six to 40 weeks after you have your baby (and ideally for life!) you try and fit in some regular cardio exercise.

Interval training Once you feel as though you have fully recovered and your baby has settled down a bit you might feel like pushing yourself a little harder, to see quicker results. This is the time to try some interval training, which will help you burn more calories in a shorter time. Try short bursts of intense exercise at RPE 8 (see page 19), for example one minute, followed by two minutes of 'ticking over' intensity, then repeat five times (or however many times you can). You can apply this to most activities including: running, gym machines, swimming and walking. For best results you really need to push yourself during your intervals – they are meant to be hard!

For very high-intensity intervals, if you are an experienced exerciser try 20 seconds of very high-intensity work followed by a ten-second rest and repeat five to ten times. This will burn some serious calories.

As with the Pregnancy Plan, for the best results you should also try to do three further moderate workouts a week for 20 to 45 minutes; this could be brisk walking, housework, cycling, gardening or anything else that fits easily into your lifestyle.

❷ EXTRAS

These are the same for the entire nine months (see the Pregnancy Plan, pages 35).

They are ab squeezes, bottom squeezes and pelvic floor exerises.

❸ RESISTANCE TRAINING
(3-Plan exercises – different for each three-month block postpartum)

For each three-month section you have a set of specifically designed resistance exercises suitable for your body in that period. The format is the same as for the Pregnancy Plan.

The only difference is that you have two sets of ab and back exercises in the first part of the New Body Plan: one set for when your abs are still recovering and to help strengthen your deep core muscles and a follow-on set for when you are ready to get back to sit-up type exercises when your diastasis has closed (these are explained on page 20!)

You will also be building on some of the exercises that you did in the Pregnancy Plan, so you may have to refer back to earlier sections if you have forgotten how to get your technique just right.

Remember to add more reps or weight or follow the harder alternatives if you feel up to working hard, but follow the basic exercises and easier options if you want a more gentle workout.

Tips See page 36.

Section 1 (weeks 0–12 postpartum)

HOW YOU MIGHT BE FEELING

What has happened?! You have bought your baby home, but what happens now? Like most parents, you are probably in an exhausted whirlwind of feeding, sleeping and coping with a crying baby, not knowing whether you are coming or going. If you are a first-time mum you are learning all the time – how to feed, change nappies without getting poo everywhere, burping and carrying your baby. But, above all, you will hopefully be feeling

happy and relieved that your new baby is finally here – safe and well. With all this going on, exercise will probably be the furthest thing from your mind, but if you can get started with some small steps as soon as possible you will reap the rewards later. You will notice that your body has changed a bit or you might not recognise it at all! It has worked very hard during pregnancy and childbirth, so you'll need to build up gradually. Your new wobbly bits and squidgy tum are only temporary – so fear not!

Summary

This is an at-a-glance summary of exercises in this section. You can refer to this once you know what you are doing rather than flicking through lots of pages each time!

Build-up plan for first six weeks. Then 6>12 weeks:

Part 1 Legs and bottom
① Back lunge and knee-lift (2 x 1kg weight)
② Wide-squat and woodchop (1 x 3kg weight)
③ Glute sweeps on all-fours
EXTRA Inner-thigh squeeze

Part 2 Upper body
① Bicep curl plus isometric hold (2 x 3kg weights)
② Narrow and wide shoulder press (2 x 1kg weights)
③ Kneeling tricep kickbacks plus tricep press-up
    (2 x 1kg)
EXTRA Chest upper back squeeze (2 x 1kg weights)

Part 3a Abs and back – Core – before diastasis (see page 20) is closed to 2cm or less
① Pelvic tilt and head-lift combo
② Superman and hold
③ Kneeling TVA
EXTRA Side-lying obliques

Part 3b Abs and back – Core – When diastasis is closed to 2cm or less
① Sit-up combo – 2 x lift, 2 x reach, 2 x across,
    2 x sides
② Weight overhead, reach to side-crunch
    (1 x 1kg weight)
③ Reverse curl
EXTRA Torso twists (2 x 3kg weight)

A rough guide for your first six weeks is outlined here. This section hardly takes up any time, meaning that you don't have to be away from your baby. If you can, get out and do some walking. Your baby will love some fresh air and walking will start getting those all-important pelvic floor and tummy muscles back into shape. This is vital as these are the muscles that have taken the biggest hit during pregnancy and childbirth. Just give these muscles a few minutes of attention a day and you'll be glad you did when you get back into exercising properly and things feel as though they are clicking back into place. Get started with the build-up plan as soon as you can and progress through the stages. You don't have to move on to the next week until you are ready, just try and do little and often. You might even have someone close by who will give you a bit of time to yourself every couple of days – this would be fantastic.

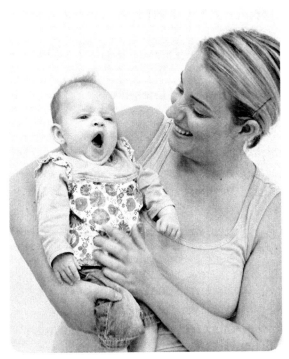

Scarlett, three months old, and Steph, 23.

Section 1 Part 1 (first six weeks)

Build-up plan for the first six weeks

Week 1 Ab pull-ins, bottom-squeezes and pelvic floor squeezes plus some walking (>30 minutes x 3 times a week).

Week 2 Ab pull-ins, bottom squeezes and pelvic floor squeezes plus some walking (>60 minutes x 3 times a week).

Week 3 As for Week 2, plus 3 x moderate cardio activity >30 minutes. Can introduce 3-Plan core abs (3a) if you are ready.

Week 4 As for Week 3. Can introduce 3-Plan arms and/or legs in addition to abs, if you are ready.

Week 5 As for Week 3/4, can increase cardio >45 minutes if you are ready.

Week 6 As for Week 5. Move on to second set of ab exercises (3b) when your diastasis is closed (see page 20) and full 6–12 weeks 3-Plan exercises when you feel up for it.

See page 35 for guidelines on ab pull-ins, bottom squeezes and pelvic floor squeezes.

Section 1 Part 2 (6–12 weeks postpartum)

PART 1 LEGS AND BOTTOM

1. Back lunge and knee-lift
(2 x 1kg weights)

Let's get cracking on getting your bottom and thighs tight and toned again! The balance required for the exercise will also start waking up your core muscles (they are still in there!)

① Hold two weights in your hands by your sides.

② Step back with one leg, with your back heel lifted and your body leaning slightly forwards. Your feet should be hip-width apart and both knees should be bent at 90 degrees. Keep your other foot still. Do not allow your front knee to go forwards beyond your toes as you lunge back.

③ As you push up and back to standing, follow through with a knee-lift on the same leg that has just lunged back and push up into a shoulder press with your hands. From here go straight back into your next lunge back, holding your tummy tight to help you balance.

Repeat 15–20 times (on each leg) and do two sets.

> **ALTERNATIVES**
> **EASIER** Just lunge backwards without the knee-lifts, no weights
> **HARDER** Bigger, deeper lunge back, higher knee-lift and hold knee-lift for a couple of seconds

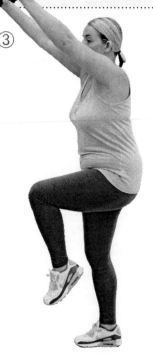

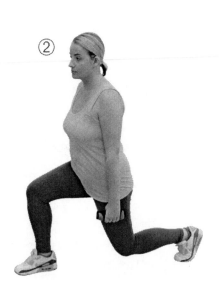

2 Wide-squat and woodchop
(1 x 3kg weight)

This fantastic exercise works your tummy and waist at the same time as all your major leg muscles. Result!

① Place a chair just behind you (optional) and stand in front of it with your feet about two hip-widths apart and toes pointed slightly out to the sides. Hold a weight in your hands, with your arms slightly bent in front of you.

② Pull in your abs and keep them tight as you bend your knees and slowly squat towards the chair, lowering the weight to just brush the floor. Keep your chin and chest lifted. Hover just above the chair (but don't sit down!).

③ Push through to lift up and begin straightening your legs. Fully extend your legs until you're back to standing position, but keep your knees soft.

④ As you push up slowly, rotate, twisting from your waist and looking over your shoulder, lifting the weight over the same shoulder. Always keep your knees in line with your toes. Come back to the starting position and repeat.

Repeat 20 times (woodchop to alternate sides) and do two sets.

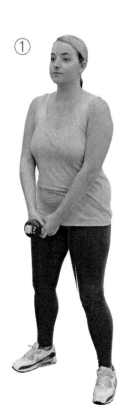

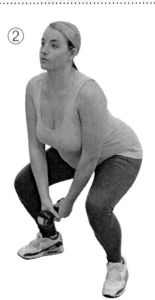

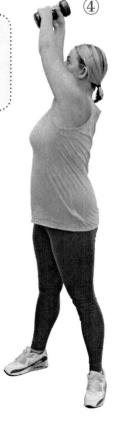

> **ALTERNATIVES**
> **EASIER** Smaller rotation, no weight, shallow squat
> **HARDER** Deeper squat, heavier weights, bigger twist and reach over shoulder

3 Glute sweeps on all-fours

This is a great one for working that wobbly bit under your bum towards the outside of your upper thigh – what woman doesn't want to tone that area up? Work it!

① With elbows on the floor, place your hands out in front of you and keep your back and neck straight.

② Extend one leg straight out behind you.

③ Cross it over the leg that is bent on the floor, so that the toe on your straight leg is just brushing the floor.

④ Slowly lift your straight leg and sweep it all the way upwards and across your body, out to the side in a semi-circle, keeping your leg straight. Squeeze your bottom and outer thigh as you lift your leg as high as you can.

⑤ Return your leg to the starting position in a returning semi-circle, keeping it off the floor if you can.

Repeat 20 times (on each leg) and do two sets.

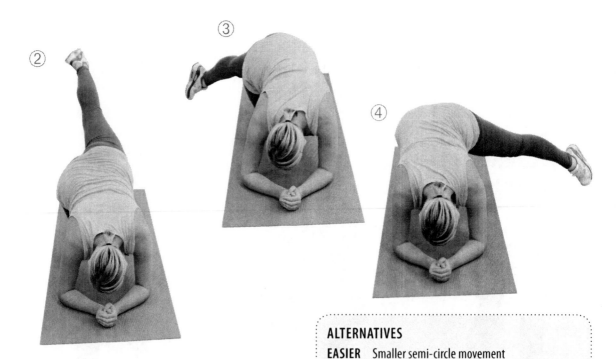

ALTERNATIVES
EASIER Smaller semi-circle movement
HARDER Larger movement – really squeeze your bottom, keeping your foot off the floor

EXTRA Inner-thigh squeeze

Focus on your inner thigh muscles as you do this exercise and make sure you can really feel them tensing.

① Sit on the floor in an upright position. Place the soles of your feet together, as close to your body as is comfortable. Your knees should be facing away from your body.

② Place your elbows on the insides of your knees and put a small amount of pressure on them.

③ As you do this squeeze upwards against the pressure with your inner thighs. Hold for a couple of seconds and release.

Repeat 15–20 times and do two sets.

ALTERNATIVES
EASIER Don't hold at the top of the move
HARDER Rest weights on your inner thighs and add resistance with your hand on both the upwards and downwards movement

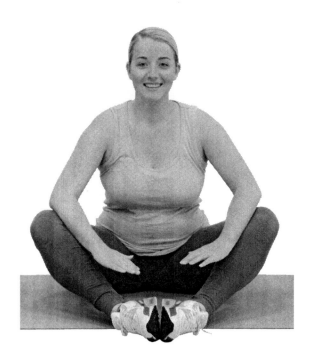

PART 2 UPPER BODY

1 Bicep curl plus isometric hold
(2 x 3kg weights)
Make sure you don't cheat by supporting the static arm at the waist or letting it drop below waist height.

① With your arms straight, hold a weight in each hand. Stand upright, with your shoulders back and abdominals pulled in. Your knees should be slightly bent.

② While you are bicep curling one arm, keep the other one completely still (in an isometric hold – how very technical!) It should be bent at 90 degrees, with the weight at waist height (the right arm is still).

③ Once you have done your reps, swap sides, without resting, to keep the biceps working.

Repeat 15–20 times (on each side) and do two sets.

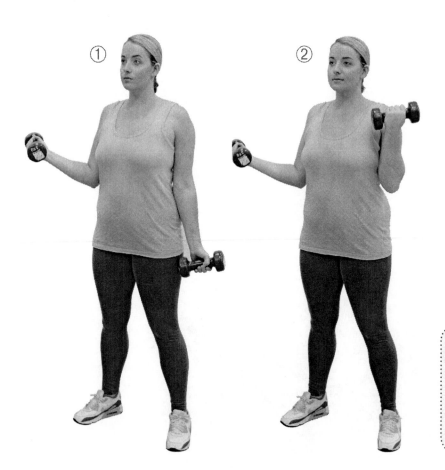

> **ALTERNATIVES**
> EASIER   Lighter weights
> HARDER   Heavier weights
>   or more reps

2 Narrow and wide shoulder press (2 x 1kg weights)

By doing two different exercises together, without a rest, you are working your upper body extra hard to get quicker results.

① Stand with your feet hip-width apart, knees soft, abdominals pulled in, shoulders back and head facing forwards.

② Hold a weight in each hand, with your arms bent and the weights at shoulder height.

③ Slowly push your arms to the sky, with your palms facing inwards. The weights should almost touch above your head.

④ Slowly lower your arms to wider than the starting position, making sure your weights don't drop below shoulder height. Again push your hands above your head, then return to start position. Alternate narrow- and wide-presses.

Repeat 15–20 times (alternating narrow and wide) and do two sets.

ALTERNATIVES
EASIER Lighter weights and/or just do narrow or wide rather than a combination
HARDER Heavier weights or more reps

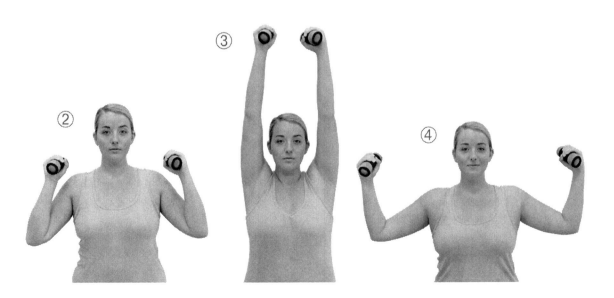

3 Kneeling tricep kickbacks plus tricep press-up (2 x 1kg weights)

Doing these two exercises together will really work those wobbly arms, so do as many as you can. The tricep press-ups will feel tough to begin with!

Tricep kickbacks

① Kneel with your knees hip-width apart. Hold a light weight in each hand, with your arms bent at 90 degrees.

② Slowly extend your arms until they are straight out behind you and squeeze your triceps. Make sure your arms stay close to your body. Bring your arms back to the starting position.

Tricep press-ups

③ Once you have done 15–20 kickbacks, lean forwards and do your tricep press-ups on the floor. These are similar to normal press-ups, but your hands should be much closer together and your elbows should bend up behind you as you dip, not out to the sides.

④ Make sure your whole body moves and your bottom lowers to the floor with each press-up.

Repeat 15–20 times (for each exercise) and do two sets.

> **ALTERNATIVES**
> EASIER   Just choose one exercise
> HARDER   Use heavier weights or try adding an extra set

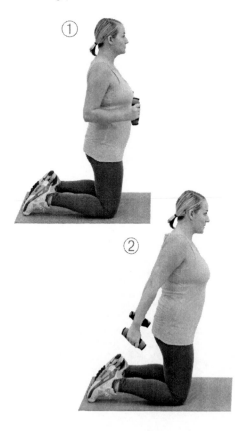

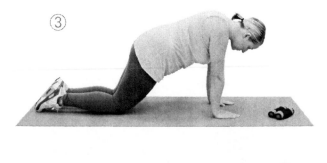

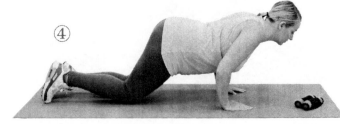

EXTRA Chest and upper-back squeeze (2 x 1kg weights)

You can do this standing or kneeling. I find it is easier to stay on your knees if you are doing this exercise straight after the tricep kickbacks.

① Hold a light weight in each hand, with your arms bent and the weights at head height. Keep your shoulders back.

② Slowly bring your arms around to the front, so that your arms touch. Keep the weights at face height.

③ Slowly return your arms to the starting position and then squeeze your upper back, bringing your shoulder blades together to take the weights slightly further around to the back.

④ Go straight back into the next chest-press without letting your weights lower.

Repeat 15–20 times and do two sets.

ALTERNATIVES
EASIER   Lighter weights
HARDER   Heavier weights or more reps

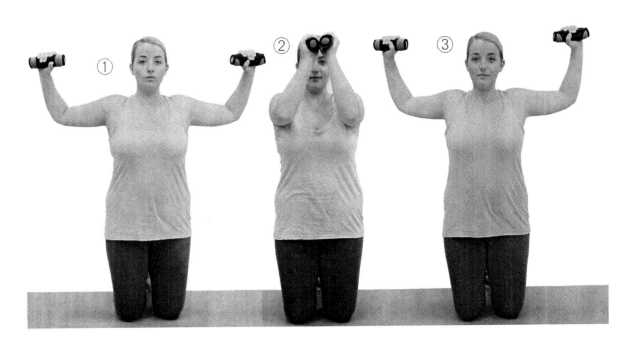

PART 3 ABS AND BACK
Before diastasis (see page 20) is closed to 2cm or less (up to six weeks)

1 Pelvic tilt and head-lift combo
By adding a pelvic tilt to the basic lift you can really draw in your deep core muscles.

① Lie on the floor, with your knees bent and the soles of your feet flat. Breathe in deeply and let your chest expand. Have your hands by your temples.

② Then, as you exhale, draw your belly button in and tilt your pelvis upwards as your draw your tummy in. Release your pelvic tilt as you lower your head to the floor.

Repeat 15–20 times and do two sets.

> **ALTERNATIVES**
> EASIER   Leave out the pelvic tilt
> HARDER   See page 46 for guidance

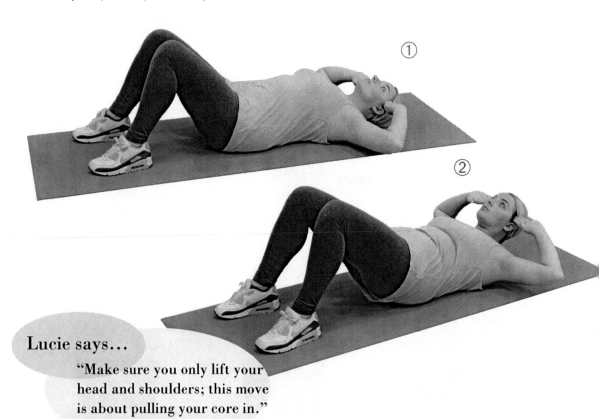

①

②

Lucie says…
"Make sure you only lift your head and shoulders; this move is about pulling your core in."

2 Superman and hold

Make sure you keep your core pulled in the whole time and keep your neck and back nice and straight.

① On your hands and knees, make sure your hands are beneath your shoulders, your knees are hip-width apart and your back and neck are straight.

② When you have pulled your tummy in, lift one leg out straight behind you and the opposite arm straight out in front of you. Keep them lifted for a couple of seconds, making your body as long as possible.

③ Once you have done your repetitions try and hold in the superman position for ten seconds on each side, keeping your core pulled in nice and tight.

Repeat 10–15 times (alternate sides then hold) and do two sets.

> **ALTERNATIVES**
> EASIER   Leave out the hold
> HARDER   Hold a light weight in the outstretched arm
> and try ankle weights

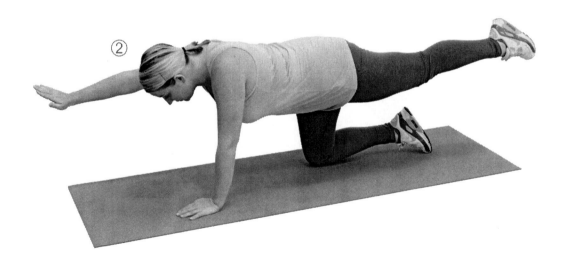

3 Kneeling ab-squeeze

Using the same principles of drawing your inner 'corset' in, which you have used before (see page 61).

① Kneel with your knees hip-width apart. Breathe in deeply and let your chest expand. Then, as you exhale, draw your belly button in. Place your hands on your hips or tummy. The rest of your body should be still.

② Hold for a couple of seconds, then breathe in as you release.

Repeat 15–20 times and do two sets.

> **ALTERNATIVES**
> HARDER   Finish with a 10-second hold-in, remembering
>   to breathe! No easy option

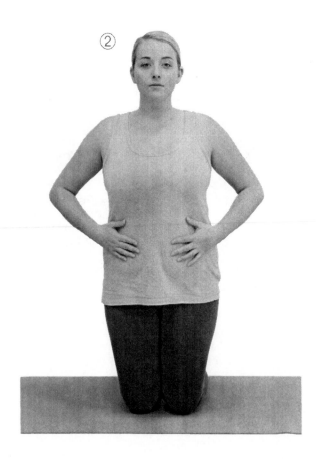

②

EXTRA Side-lying obliques

If you struggle to get your head and shoulders comfortable, put a pillow under your head

① Lie on your side with your knees bent behind you at 90 degrees.

② Breathe in deeply and let your chest expand. Then, as you exhale, draw your belly button in. Place your hands wherever they are most comfortable. The rest of your body should be still. Hold for a couple of seconds, then breathe in as you release. Pull in your side abdominals, too.

Repeat 15–20 times (on each side) and do two sets.

ALTERNATIVES

HARDER   Finish with a 10-second hold-in, remembering to breathe! No easy option

---

②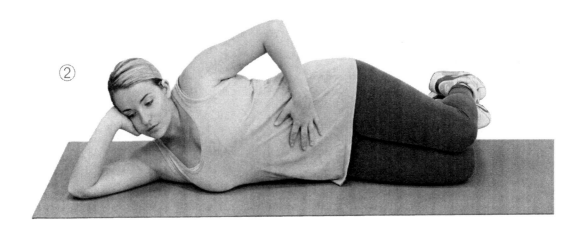

PART 3 ABS AND BACK

Core – When diastasis is closed to 2cm or less (around six weeks).

1 Sit-up combo – 2 x lift, 2 x reach, 2 x across, 2 x sides

Doing these different types of sit-up will work your tummy muscles in lots of ways, encouraging them back to flatness!

① Lie back on the floor with your knees bent and the soles of your feet flat. Breathe in deeply and let your chest expand. Then, as you exhale, draw your belly button in and tilt your pelvis upwards slightly so that your lower back touches the floor or you have a small natural arch.

② Place your hands by your temples. Gradually lift your head and shoulders off the floor towards the ceiling, breathing out as you do and focusing on pulling your abs in. The rest of your body should be still. There should be a gap between your chin and your chest. Take care not to pull on your neck.

③ Breathe in as you lower back down. A photo of the basic head lift is shown in the Pregnancy Plan, Trimester 1 (see page 46).

④ Do two normal lifts followed by two reaching your hands to your knees.

⑤ Follow with two reaching across to the opposite knee

⑥ Follow with two reaching down to each side. Make sure that you keep your chin off your chest at all times.

Repeat five times (all eight lifts) and do two sets.

> **ALTERNATIVES**
> **EASIER** Choose one or two rather than all four moves
> **HARDER** Hold light hand weights or do eight repetitions of each rather than two

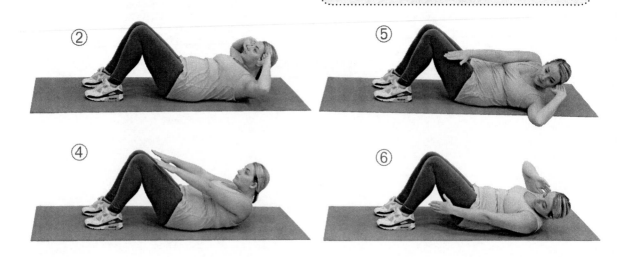

2 Weight overhead, reach to side-crunch (1 x 1kg weight)

By bringing a weight into your tummy exercises you add extra resistance for fantastic results. You can support your neck with your hand if you like.

① Lie on the floor with your legs out straight and your heels on the floor. Breathe in deeply and let your chest expand. Then as you exhale draw your belly button in and tilt your pelvis upwards so that your lower back touches the floor or you have a small natural arch.

② Place one hand by your temples and a weight in the other hand stretched out above your head.

③ Gradually lift your head and shoulders off the floor towards the ceiling, breathing out as you do and focusing on pulling your abs in.

④ As you lift your head, bring one knee in towards your chest and reach the weight down to your side, on the same side as the knee that is coming in.

⑤ Breathe in as you lower back down to position 2. Do all your repetitions on one side before swapping.

Repeat 15–20 times (on each side) and do two sets.

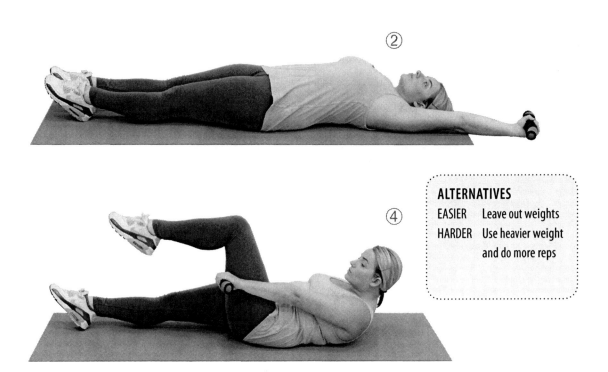

② ④

ALTERNATIVES

EASIER   Leave out weights

HARDER   Use heavier weight and do more reps

3 Reverse curl

This exercise is great for your lower tummy area – that extra tummy flab won't be there forever!

① Lie back on the floor with your knees at 90 degrees. Draw your belly button in and tilt your pelvis upwards slightly so that your lower back touches the floor or you have a small natural arch. Place your hands by your sides.

② Gradually lift knees towards your chest, breathing out as you do so and focusing on pulling your lower abs in.

③ Breathe in as you lower back down to the starting position.

Repeat 15–20 times and do two sets.

ALTERNATIVES

EASIER   Have your legs nearer the floor and make a smaller movement

HARDER   Have a light weight between your knees. Try holding your legs in position when they are curled in

---

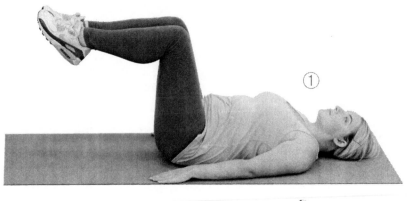

①

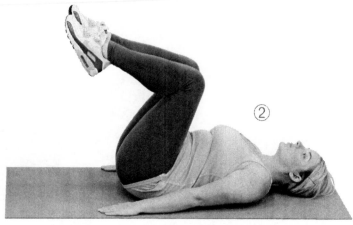

②

EXTRA Torso twists (2 x 3kg weights)

Make sure your hips face forwards at all times and imagine you are wearing your tightest skinny jeans – zip those abs up! This will work you arms, too.

① Hold a weight in each hand, with your arms comfortably in front of your chest and the weights together. Stand upright, with your shoulders back and abdominals pulled in. Your knees should be slightly bent.

② Twist from your waist so that your weights move around to one side. Come back to centre then twist to the other side.

Repeat 50 times (alternate sides) and do two sets.

ALTERNATIVES
EASIER Don't use any weights.
HARDER Add a punch across your body as you twist, or do more reps. Try some fast twists, too!

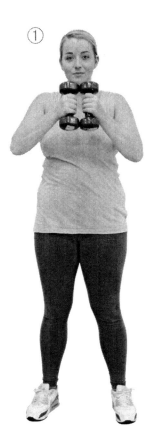

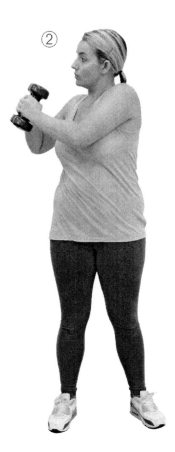

Section 2 (weeks 13–26 postpartum)

HOW YOU MIGHT BE FEELING

Hopefully life will be settling down for you a bit by now! You will feel more confident about taking your baby out and about, changing nappies and doing general baby things. You should also be getting a bit more sleep (I hope!) and your little one will be brightening up your whole day by giving you a beaming smile! He or she is starting to look more like a little person and less like a tiny baby (where does the time go?)

You might find it harder to exercise now that your baby is awake more during the day. If this is the case then just fit it in whenever you can, even if it is in ten-minute chunks throughout the day. Perhaps you can ask someone to give you a little bit of time off; you can stay close by and even exercise near to your baby if you like.

Your body should be starting to return to its pre-pregnancy state, but this happens at different rates for different people, so fear not if you aren't back into your skinny jeans yet. Here is a whole new set of exercises to work you harder, to continue to pull everything back into place.

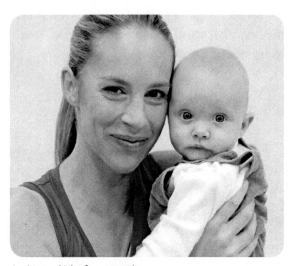

Jo, 31, and Isla, four months.

Summary

This is an at-a-glance summary of exercises in this section. You can refer to it once you know what you are doing rather than flicking through lots of pages each time!

Part 1 Legs and bottom
① Forward lunge and side-squat (2 x 1kg)
② Figure-of-eight squat (1 x 3kg)
③ Three-point bottom-squeeze
EXTRA 1 leg-squat plus shoulder push (2 x 1kg)

Part 2 Upper body
① Hammer curl plus isometric hold (2 x 3kg)
② Mack-raise (2x 1kg)

③ Tricep bridge and roll-back
EXTRA Chest-flies on all-fours (2 x 1kg)

Part 3 Abs and back
① Weight overhead, sit-up straight arms and leg (1x 1kg)
② Sit-up and twist and punch (2 x 1kg)
③ Slow elbows to knees
EXTRA Scissor legs (1 x 3kg)

PLUS: Plank for 30 seconds and >50 x pelvic tilt and head-lift combo

PART 1 LEGS AND BOTTOM

1 Forward lunge and side-squat
(2 x 1 kg weights)

You have done lunges and squats before; now combine the two for excellent results.

① Firstly to lunge, step forwards with one leg so that the other back heel comes off the floor and lower your upper body down, bending your legs (don't step out too far). Your feet should be a hip-width apart and both knees should be bent at 90 degrees. Keep your upper body upright, with shoulders back and don't lean forwards. Do not allow your front knee to go forwards beyond your toes as you come down. Bicep curl as you lunge

② Push up and back to standing. A picture of the basic lunge is shown in the Pregnancy Plan, Trimester 1 (see page 38).

③ Next, on the same leg and without resting your foot on the floor (just tap the toe) side-step into a deep side-lunge, pushing your bottom backwards, with your toes pointing slightly outwards and your chin and chest lifted. Push your arms forwards.

④ Push back to standing tall and go straight into your next forward lunge on the same leg. Do all your reps on one leg before moving on to the other side.

Repeat 20 times (alternate lunge and squat) and do two sets (on each leg).

> **ALTERNATIVES**
> **EASIER** Shallow lunges and squats, leave out the arms, just do one of the two exercises
> **HARDER** Use heavier weights, deeper lunges and squats and add a set of 10 deep lunge and/or squat pulses at the end

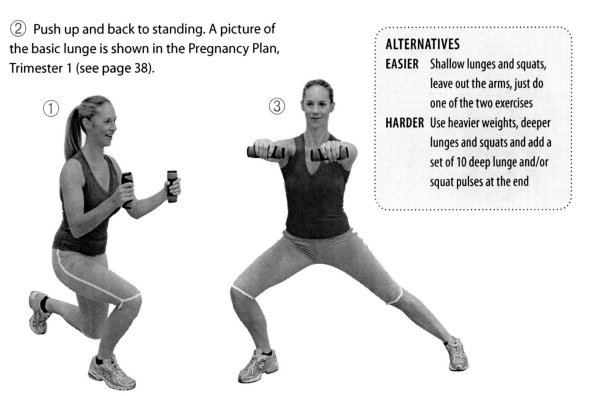

2 Figure-of-eight squat (1 x 3kg weight)

Using the weight makes you work harder than for a normal squat and it gets your arms involved – burn that fat!

① Hold a weight in one hand with your arm out at 90 degrees. Stand with your feet just over hip-width apart and toes pointed slightly out.

② Pull in your abs and keep them tight as you bend your knees and slowly squat. Keep your chin and chest lifted.

③ As you squat, pass your weight through your legs to the other hand in a figure of eight.

④ Push through to lift up and begin straightening your legs. Fully extend the legs

until you're back to standing position, but keep your knees soft.

⑤ As you push up, bring your other arm up to 90 degrees, now holding the weight out to the other side.

Repeat 20 times (passing the weight alternate ways) and do two sets.

> **ALTERNATIVES**
> **EASIER** No weights, shallow squat, don't include figure of eight.
> **HARDER** Deeper squat, heavier weight, try holding the squat in the lowest position and passing the weight through in a figure of eight ten times, keeping your legs still (isometric)

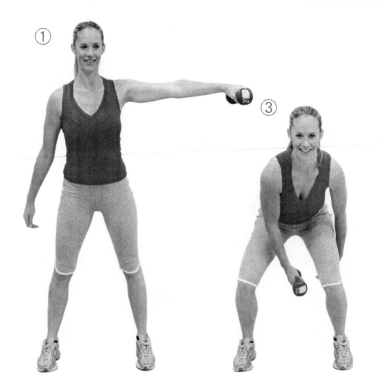

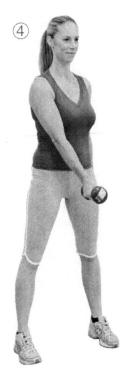

3 Three-point bottom-squeeze

This exercise will really tone your bottom – don't rest between positions!

① On all-fours on the floor, rest on your forearms, looking down at the floor. Extend one leg out behind you, with your foot flexed. Push your leg up to the ceiling, squeezing your bottom as you do so.

② Return to the starting position, keeping your toe just off the floor, if you can. Do ten reps with your leg straight out behind you, ten reps with your leg out at a 45-degree angle to the side and ten reps with your leg out to the side, as close as you can get to a 90-degree angle. When your leg is out to the side you will need to come up on to your hands, not your forearms.

Repeat 30 times (ten in each of the three positions on each leg) and do two sets.

> **ALTERNATIVES**
> **EASIER** Just stick with normal bottom squeezes with you leg out behind you.
> **HARDER** Finish with a set of 20 high pulses with your leg at the top of the movement (straight out behind you), add ankle weights, more reps at each point.

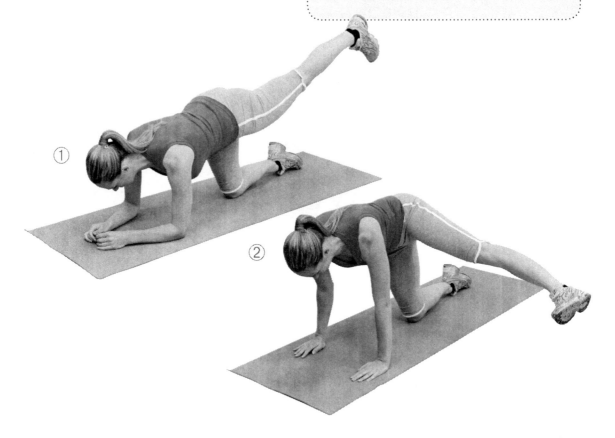

EXTRA One leg-squat and shoulder push (2 x 3kg weights)

All your weight needs to be on your back leg; your front toe should just 'kiss' the floor, purely to give you a bit of balance.

① Hold a weight in each hand with your hands in front of your shoulders. Stand with your feet a hip-width apart, with one toe pointing forwards.

② Slowly, bend your front knee, squatting down. Go as low as you can, then push back up to the starting position.

③ Push through to lift up and begin straightening your back leg. Fully extend the leg until you're back to standing, squeezing your bottom in the top position.

④ As you push up push your weights upwards into a shoulder push. Come back to the starting position and repeat.

Repeat 20 times and do two sets.

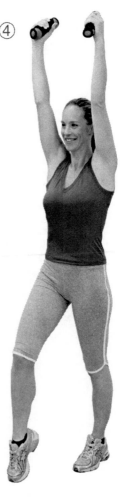

ALTERNATIVES
EASIER Lighter weights, leave out the shoulder push, shallow squat, hands on hips
HARDER Deeper squat, heavier weights, finish with set of low pulse one leg squats

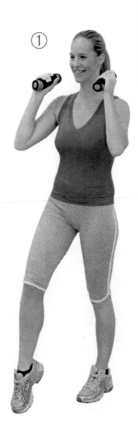
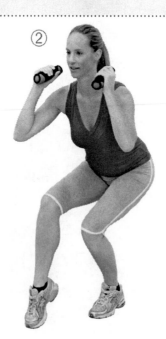

PART 2 UPPER BODY

1 Hammer curl plus isometric hold (2 x 3kg weights)

Make sure you don't cheat by supporting the static arm at the waist or letting it drop below waist height.

① With your arms straight, hold a weight in each hand. Stand upright, with your shoulders back and abdominals pulled in. Your knees should be slightly bent.

② Do your hammer curls with one arm at a time. Hammers are basically bicep curls with your palms facing inwards. Keep the curl nice and close to your body. While you are curling one arm keep the other one completely still. It should be bent at 90 degrees, with the weight at waist height. Once you have done your reps, swap sides, without resting, to keep your biceps working.

Repeat 15–20 times (on each side) and do two sets.

Option: add tricep kickback after each hammer curl (see page 56).

①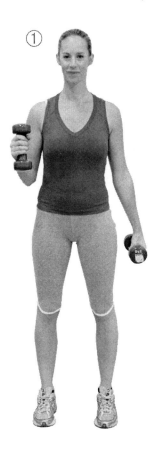

②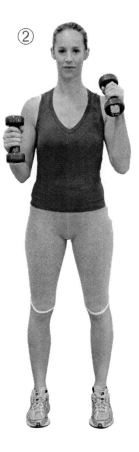

ALTERNATIVES
EASIER   Lighter weights, less reps
HARDER   Heavier weights, finish with a set of 20 normal hammer curls straight after your set using both arms

2 Mack-raise (2 x 1kg weights)

These are fab for toning your arms and shoulders – these are probably getting a lot of work carrying your little one plus a massive changing bag around!

① Hold a light weight in each hand, with your arms slightly bent down by your sides. Stand upright with your shoulders back and abdominals pulled in. Your knees should be slightly bent.

② Slowly raise one arm up, forwards from your sides to 90 degrees into a front-raise and raise the other arm up sideways into a side-raise at the same time. Don't raise them above shoulder height. Hold for a couple of seconds, then drop your arms back to your sides.

③ On the next rep your other arm comes forwards, while the opposite one lifts out to the side. Make sure your hips stay solid and facing forwards.

Repeat 15–20 times (alternate sides) and do two sets.

> **ALTERNATIVES**
> **EASIER** Lighter or no weights, less reps
> **HARDER** Heavier weights, more reps

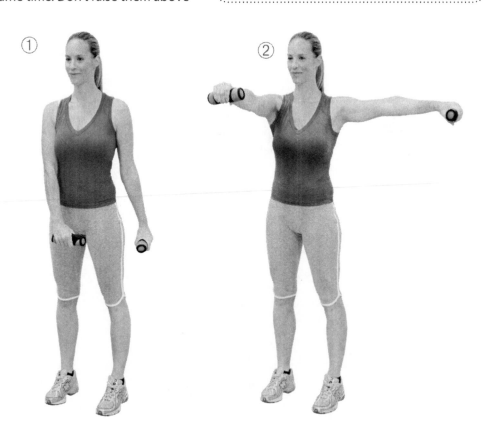

3 Tricep bridge and roll-back

No excuses for jelly underarms after doing these two exercises together – think of those strappy tops!

Tricep bridge

① Sit on the floor with your feet flat and a hip-width apart and your hands beside you, facing forwards (it is very important that your hands face forwards, towards your toes).

② Lift your bottom up.

③ Do a dip by slowly lowering your body to the floor and pushing back up through the triceps, making sure your elbows do not drift out to the sides.

Roll-back

④ Once you have done 15–20 dips, without resting, sit down on the floor then lean back, supporting your weight. Push back up, using your triceps. Make sure throughout the roll-back that your chest stays lifted and your hands stay close to your body and facing forwards.

Repeat 15–20 times (for each exercise) and do two sets.

> **ALTERNATIVES**
> **EASIER**   Just do one of the two exercises, shallow dips and small roll-backs
> **HARDER** Deep dips and roll-back, finish with hold at lowest point of roll-back for ten seconds – you might shake!

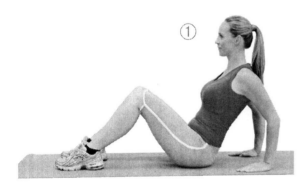

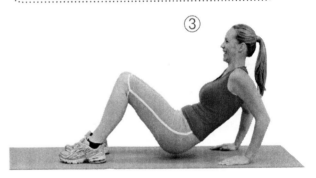

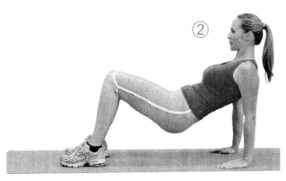

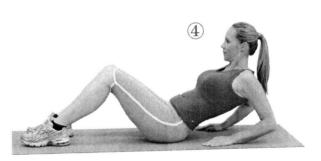

EXTRA Chest-flies on all-fours (2x 1kg weights)

Really squeeze your shoulder blades together as you lift the weight out to the side – think of that lovely toned back.

① On all-fours on the floor, place your hands on the floor beneath your shoulders and keep your back and neck straight. Hold a light weight in each hand.

② Slowly lift one arm up and out to the side, squeezing your back as you do so. Your elbow should be slightly soft.

③ Slowly lower the weight back to the starting position.

Repeat 15–20 times (on each side) and do two sets.

> **ALTERNATIVES**
> **EASIER** Lighter weights, less reps
> **HARDER** Heavier weights, more reps

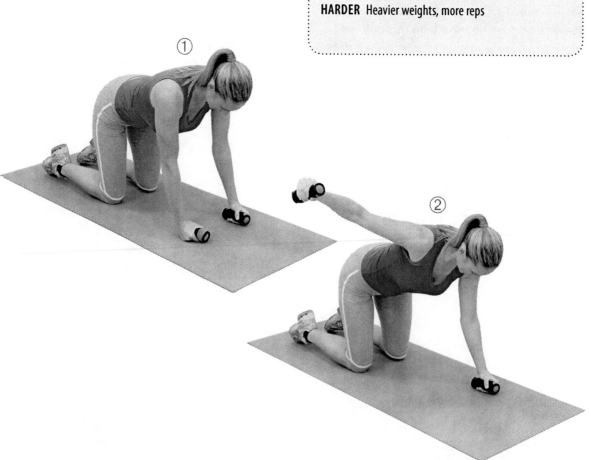

PART 3 ABS AND BACK

1 Weight overhead, sit up, straight arms and leg (1x 1kg weight)

Don't cheat by bringing your leg too far up – remember that your tummy should be doing all the work.

① Lie back on the floor with your legs out straight and your heels on the floor. Breathe in deeply and let your chest expand. Then, as you exhale, draw your belly button in and tilt your pelvis upwards slightly so that your lower back touches the floor or you have a small natural arch. Stretch your hands out above your head, holding a light weight.

② Gradually lift your head and shoulders off the floor towards the ceiling, breathing out as you do so, focusing on pulling your abs in. As you lift your head, lift one leg, keeping it fairly straight and reach the weight up to your toe.

③ Breathe in as you lower back down to the starting position, with the weight above your head. Do the next rep with the other leg.

Repeat 15–20 times (alternate legs) and do two sets.

ALTERNATIVES
EASIER No weight, hands by temples, leave out leg, head and shoulder lifts only (see page 90)
HARDER Heavier weight, more reps, finish with 20 pulses at top point reaching up towards your toes. Keep your chin lifted at all times!

2 Sit-up and twist and punch
(2 x 1kg weights)

Really try and turn to each side as you punch, to work your waist effectively.

① Lie back on the floor with your knees bent and the soles of your feet flat. Breathe in deeply and let your chest expand. Then as you exhale, draw your belly button in and tilt your pelvis upwards slightly, so that your lower back touches the floor or you have a small natural arch either side of your chest.

② Gradually lift your head and shoulders off the floor towards the ceiling, breathing out as you do so, focusing on pulling your abs in. The rest of your body should be still. There should be a gap between your chin and your chest and take care not to pull on your neck.

③ Keep your tummy strong and hold it still as you twist and punch to each side.

④ Come back to centre and breathe in as you lower back down. As you do so roll back one vertebrae at a time in a controlled descent.

Repeat 10–15 times (punching both sides) and do two sets.

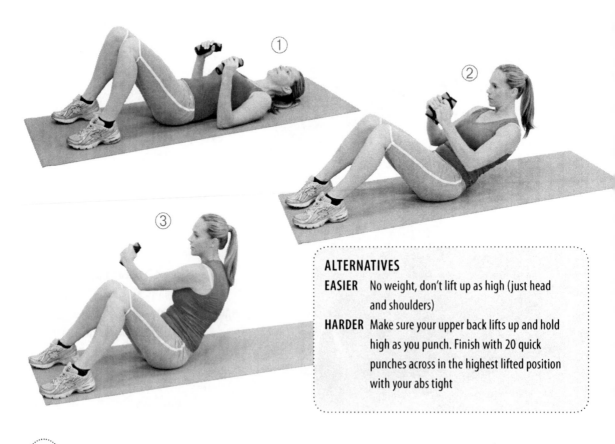

ALTERNATIVES

EASIER No weight, don't lift up as high (just head and shoulders)

HARDER Make sure your upper back lifts up and hold high as you punch. Finish with 20 quick punches across in the highest lifted position with your abs tight

3 Slow elbows to knees

The slower you go and the straighter and closer you can get your legs to the floor the more you will be working your abs.

① Lie back on the floor with your knees bent and the soles of your feet flat on the floor. Breathe in deeply and let your chest expand. Then as you exhale draw your belly button in and tilt your pelvis upwards slightly so that your lower back touches the floor or you have a small natural arch. Have your hands by your temples.

② Gradually lift your head and shoulders off the floor towards the ceiling, breathing out as you do so and focusing on pulling your abs in. There should be a gap between your chin and your chest. Take care not to pull on your neck.

③ Bring your knees up into a crunch position.

④ Lean across (hands still by your temples) so that one elbow touches (or nearly touches) the opposite knee. The other leg should be extended. Then swap, so that the other leg is extended and the other elbow and knee touch. Continue in a slow, controlled cycling motion (count to four each side).

Repeat 20–30 times (alternate legs) and do two sets.

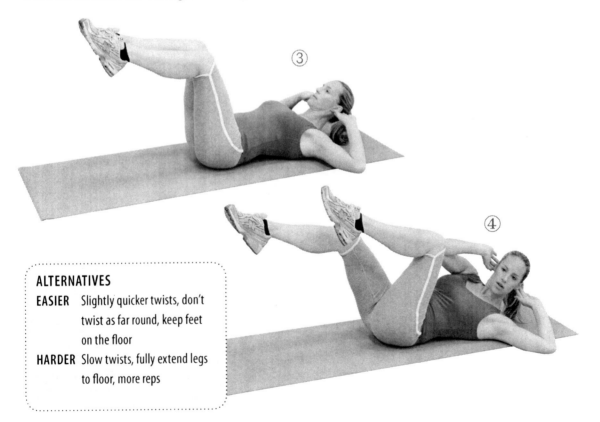

ALTERNATIVES

EASIER Slightly quicker twists, don't twist as far round, keep feet on the floor

HARDER Slow twists, fully extend legs to floor, more reps

EXTRA Scissor legs (1 x 3kg weight)

As you become stronger, see if you can scissor your legs just above the floor. The lower you go the harder your lower abs will work. If you want to go crazy, mix it up and scissor sideways as well!

① Lie back on the floor with your knees bent and the soles of your feet flat on the floor. Breathe in deeply and let your chest expand. Then as you exhale draw your belly button in and tilt your pelvis upwards slightly so that your lower back touches the floor or you have created a small natural arch. Place your hands by your sides.

② Bring your legs up to a 45–90-degree angle to begin with and push your arms forwards.

③ Lower one leg to the floor (as close as you can), then return it to the starting position, lowering the other leg as you do so.

④ Continue in a slow, controlled scissor motion. As you scissor your legs pass your weight from hand to hand between your legs in a figure of eight.

Repeat 20–30 times (alternate legs) and do two sets.

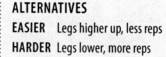

ALTERNATIVES
EASIER Legs higher up, less reps
HARDER Legs lower, more reps

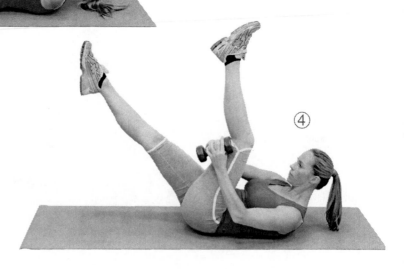

PLUS (as often as possible!)
- Plank for 30 seconds
- >50 x pelvic tilt and head-lift combo
  (see page 90)

The plank

① To do the plank, lift your body, resting on your forearms and toes. Keep your back and neck straight and bottom down (it has a tendency to stick up!)

② Hold your abs in tightly and keep as still as possible. Give this a miss if you have high blood pressure.

③ If you find it too challenging on your toes, simply drop to your knees, keeping your abs in tight and bottom nice and low.

①

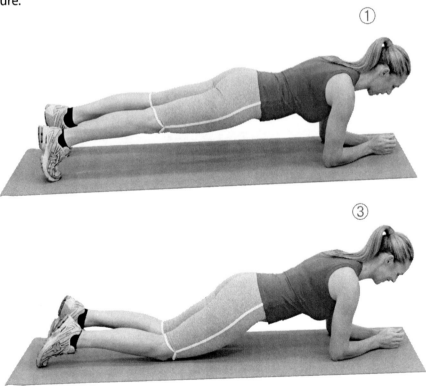

③

111

Section 3 (weeks 27–40 postpartum)

HOW YOU MIGHT BE FEELING

A lot has changed in the past few weeks. Your baby has been a charming, cooing little lovely for the last couple of months – and she hasn't started running around and causing trouble – yet. Make the most of this slightly more manageable state of affairs!

We are on the home stretch with the New Body Plan now! You have done incredibly well to stick with the 3-Plan, so keep going! Even if you think your body is back in shape, try to carry on because it could be even better than before you had your baby! You also need to maintain your fitness levels. Try and push yourself in this section – do a couple of extra reps or increase your weights. Now your body has more or less fully recovered from pregnancy and birth, you can continue with slightly more challenging exercises to see rapid changes in muscle tone and tummy flatness. Go for it!

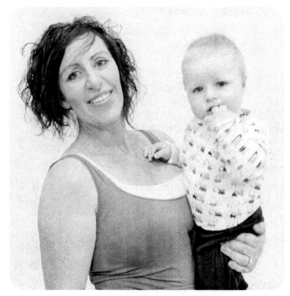

Simone, 42, mum of three, and Wilbur, 8 months.

Summary

This is an at-a-glance summary of exercises in this section. You can refer to this once you know what you are doing rather than flicking through lots of pages each time!

Part 1 Legs and bottom
① Plié squat and overhead reach (2 x 3kg)
② Diagonal and lunge and punch (2 x 1kg)
③ Jump-squat
EXTRA Standing hip extension

Part 2 Upper body
① Tricep overhead press (1 x 3kg)
② Half-arnold shoulder press (2 x 3kg)
③ All-fours row (2 x 3kg)
EXTRA Around-the-world (2 x 1kg)

Part 3 Abs and back
① Double crunch (2 x 1kg)
② Roll-back weight overhead (1 x 1kg)
③ Straight leg oblique cross with weight (1 x 1kg)
EXTRA Back extension

PLUS Plank for >60 seconds and >100 x pelvic tilt and head lift combo. Work your abs even harder.

PART 1 LEGS AND BOTTOM

1 Plié-squat and overhead reach
(2 x 3kg weights)

Adding weight and a reach to the basic plié-squat will work even more muscles in one exercise.

① Stand with your feet two to three hip-widths apart, your toes pointing outwards. Hold a weight in each hand at shoulder height.

② Pull in your abs and keep them tight as you bend your knees and slowly squat, keeping your back straight and shoulders back. Your bottom should not push backwards.

③ Hold in the lowest position for a couple of seconds, then fully extend your legs until you're back to the starting position, but keep your knees soft.

④ As you push (keeping your hands wide) back up, extend your arms over your head. Lower the weights back to your shoulders as you move straight into your next squat.

Repeat 20 times and do two sets.

> **ALTERNATIVES**
> **EASIER** Shallow squats, leave out the arms (hands on hips instead)
> **HARDER** Use heavier weights, deeper squats and add a set of 20 deep plié-squats pulses at the end

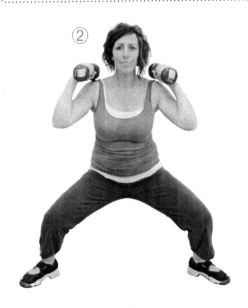

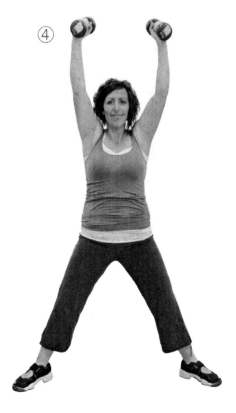

2 Diagonal and lunge and punch (2 x 1kg weights)

Doing your lunges out to the corners will work your leg muscles in a slightly different way and make you use your core muscles to balance.

① Hold a weight in each hand, with your hands in front of your shoulders.

② To lunge, step out to 45 degrees with one leg, so that the other back heel comes off the floor, and lower your upper body down, bending your legs (don't step out too far). Don't cross your feet (your right leg comes out 45 degrees to your right side). Your knees should be bent at 90 degrees. Keep your upper body upright, with shoulders back and don't lean forwards. Don't allow your front knee to go forwards beyond your toes as you come down.

③ As you lunge, punch the opposite arm across your body at chest height. Come back to the starting position and repeat.

Repeat 15–20 times (one side at a time) and do two sets.

ALTERNATIVES
EASIER No weights, leave out the punch, lunge forwards rather than diagonal
HARDER Deeper lunge, heavier weight

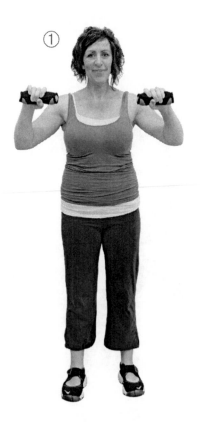

①

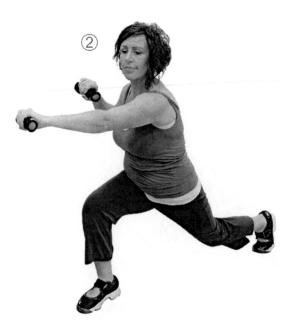

②

3 Jump-squat

Jump as high as you can and squat as low as you can to make this exercise really work for you!

① Stand with your feet about a hip-width apart. Pull in your abs and keep them tight as you bend your knees and slowly squat down, dropping your hands to the floor.

② From the squat position, push up into a jump and extend your arms above your head, jumping off the floor.

③ From your jump, slowly lower into your next squat without resting.

Repeat 15–20 times and do two sets.

> **ALTERNATIVES**
> **EASIER** Normal squats with no jump
> **HARDER** Very deep squat and very high jump – reach for the sky!

②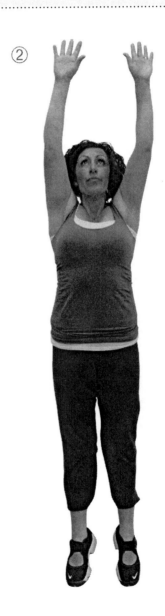

①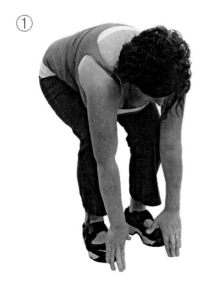

115

EXTRA Standing hip extension

Pretend you are cracking a nut at the top of your leg, under your bottom as you lift!

Repeat 20 times (one side at a time) and do two sets. Keep the rest of your body still, isolating your bottom muscles.

① Stand with your feet a hip-width apart and hands on hips. Lean slightly forwards from your waist and get your balance.

② From here, lift one leg behind you, keeping it as straight as you can, squeezing your bottom as you lift. Hold for a second then return to the starting position and repeat.

> **ALTERNATIVES**
> **EASIER** Hold on to a wall or chair, lower lifts
> **HARDER** Finish with a set of 20 pulses with your bottom squeezed as tight as you can, add an ankle weight

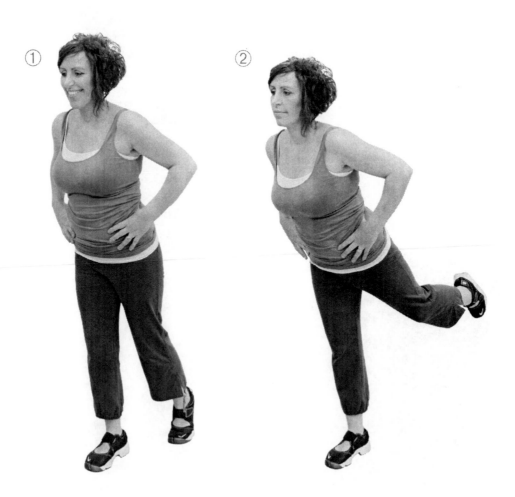

PART 3 UPPER BODY

1 Tricep overhead press (1x 3kg weight)

Make sure you don't let your elbows drift out to the sides – keep them nice and close to your head.

① Hold a weight in your hands with your arms above your head. Stand upright, with your shoulders back and abdominals pulled in. Your knees should be slightly bent.

② Slowly drop the weight behind your head in a controlled manner, then push it back up to the starting position, making sure you keep your elbows narrow. Keep the rest of your body still and your chin lifted. Focus on squeezing your tricep as you press up.

Repeat 15–20 times and do two sets.

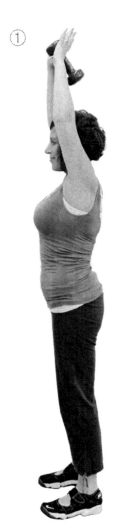

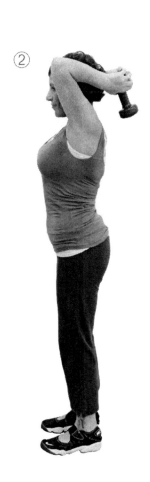

> **ALTERNATIVES**
> **EASIER** Lighter weight, less reps
> **HARDER** Heavier weight, more reps

2 Half-arnold shoulder press
(2x 3kg weights)

Another fab exercise for your upper arms – make sure your palms face you at all times.

① Stand with your feet a hip-width apart, knees soft, abdominals pulled in, shoulders back and head facing forwards. Hold a weight in each hand, with your arms bent and the weights at head height.

② Slowly push your arms to the sky, with your palms facing towards you. The weights should still be parallel as you push up and they should not meet at the top.

③ Slowly lower your arms to the starting position, making sure your weights don't drop below head height.

Repeat 15–20 times and do two sets.

ALTERNATIVES
EASIER   Lighter weights, less reps
HARDER   Heavier weights, more reps

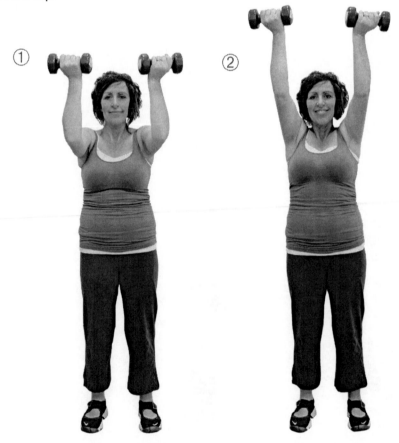

3 All-fours row (2x 3kg weights)

Really squeeze your shoulder blades together as you squeeze up to tone your upper back.

① On your hands and knees, make sure your hands are under your shoulders, your knees are a hip-width apart and your back and neck are straight. Hold a weight in each hand. Hold your tummy in, but remember to breathe comfortably.

② Take one hand out slightly in front of you so your arm is straighter. Strongly bring this hand up to your waist, squeezing your upper back. Return to the starting position and repeat.

Repeat 10–15 times (on each side) and do two sets. Do all reps on one side first.

> **ALTERNATIVES**
> **EASIER** Lighter weights
> **HARDER** Heavier weights, more reps

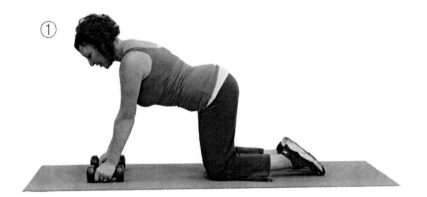

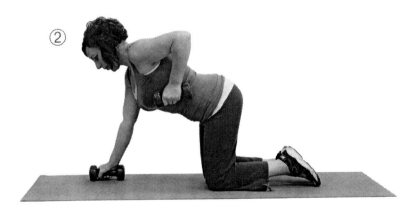

119

EXTRA Around-the-world
(2 x 1kg weights)

Not only is this exercise a cheesy song by East 17 (remember them?), it's another great one for working lots of upper-body muscles all in one go.

① Stand with your feet a hip-width apart, knees soft, abdominals pulled in, shoulders back and head facing forwards. Hold a weight in each hand, with your arms behind your back, your palms facing upwards and the weights just at the top of your bottom.

② and ③ Slowly take the weights out to your sides and up to the sky in front of you, so that they touch. This move should be a big arm circle and it should be controlled, so definitely don't swing your arms.

④ Slowly return your arms to the starting position, circling them back through the same path. Keep the rest of your body still and your chin lifted.

Repeat 15–20 times and do two sets.

> **ALTERNATIVES**
> **EASIER**   Lighter or no weights, less reps
> **HARDER**   Heavier weights, more reps

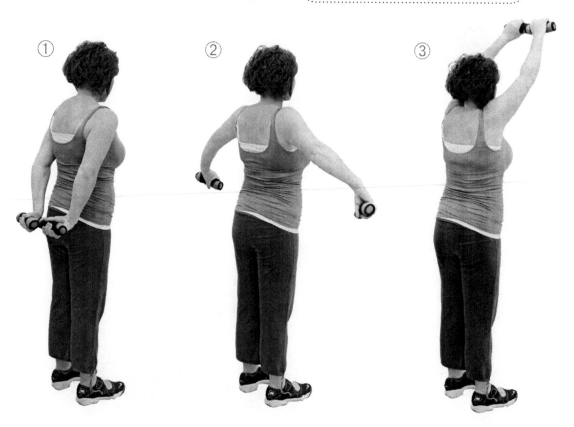

PART 3 ABS AND BACK

1 Double crunch with weights (2 x 1 kg weights)

Make sure you focus the whole time on drawing your abs in as you squeeze up and don't forgot to breathe!

① Lie back on the floor with your knees bent and lifted to 90 degrees. Hold a light weight in each hand by your temples.

② Gradually lift your head, shoulders and upper back off the floor towards the ceiling, breathing out as you do so. At the same time bring your knees in, squeezing your lower abdominals and reach your weights towards your toes. There should be a gap between your chin and your chest. Breathe in as you lower back down and repeat. Make sure you don't knee yourself in the face!

Repeat 15–20 times and do two sets.

> **ALTERNATIVES**
> **EASIER** No weights (or one weight on your chest if you want to support your neck with one hand), just choose the top half or bottom half rather than combining the two
> **HARDER** More reps, finish with a set of 20 pulses at the highest point

①
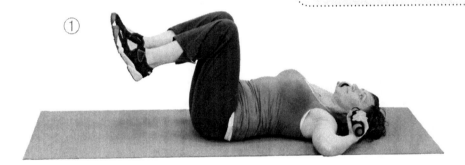

②
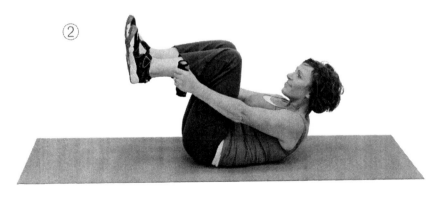

2 Roll-back weight overhead (1x 1kg weights)

Try to feel each individual vertebrae rolling down on to the floor, one at a time. If this is a bit tough to begin with, then leave the weight out at first.

① Sit upright, with your knees bent and your heels on the floor. Breathe in deeply and let your chest expand. Then as you exhale draw your belly button in so that you have engaged your core.

② Stretch your hands out, bringing them over your head, holding a light weight. Gradually roll backwards on the mat, keeping your tummy pulled in tight and your arms straight. Slowly and gradually let your spine uncurl on to the floor. Tap the weight on the floor behind your head (if you can!).

③ Curl your spine back up to the starting position in the same controlled manner as you descended.

Repeat 15–20 times and do two sets.

ALTERNATIVES

EASIER No weight, hands on knees, head and shoulder lifts if you don't like the rolls

HARDER Heavier weight, focus on rolling your spine to the floor with your abs in even more slowly

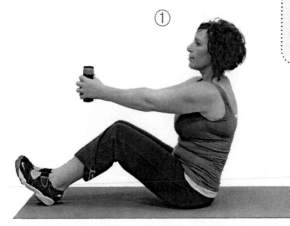

①

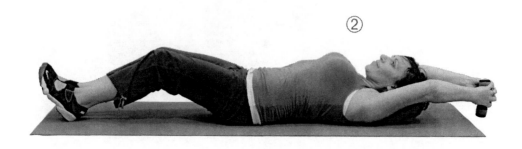

②

3 Straight-leg oblique cross with weight (1x 1kg weight)

Remember: this exercise should be working your waist, so make sure that all the effort comes from your tum rather than your arms or legs.

① Lie back on the floor with your legs out wide and straight and your heels on the floor. Breathe in deeply and let your chest expand. Then as you exhale, draw your belly button in and tilt your pelvis upwards slightly so that your lower back touches the floor or you have a small natural arch.

② Have one hand stretched out wide above your head, holding a light weight, and the other out to the side.

③ Gradually lift your head and shoulders off the floor towards the ceiling, focusing on pulling your abs in. As you lift your head, raise one leg, keeping it fairly straight and reach up with the opposite arm (the one holding the weight!) up to your toe.

④ Breathe in as you lower back down to the starting position. Do all your reps on one side before swapping.

Repeat 15–20 times (on each side) and do two sets.

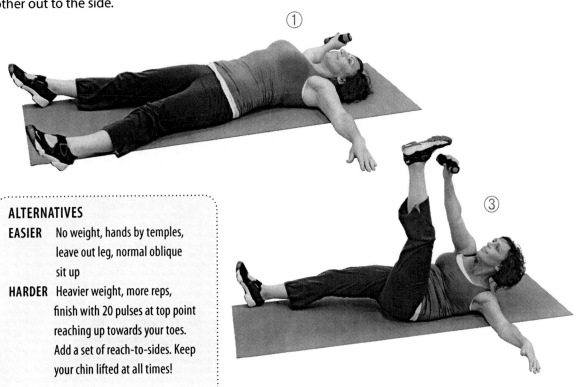

① ③

ALTERNATIVES

EASIER No weight, hands by temples, leave out leg, normal oblique sit up

HARDER Heavier weight, more reps, finish with 20 pulses at top point reaching up towards your toes. Add a set of reach-to-sides. Keep your chin lifted at all times!

EXTRA Back extension

This exercise will work your lower back to complement the tummy work and keep the dreaded back muffin top at bay.

① Lie on your front with your toes stretched out and your legs about a hip-width apart. Have your hands by your temples.

② Slowly lift your head and shoulders off the floor, squeezing your lower back. Make sure your neck remains straight and level with your spine. Only come up as far as is comfortable.

③ Slowly lower to the starting position. If you find this a bit tough to begin with, then start with your forearms resting on the floor as you lift up.

Repeat 15–20 times and do two sets.

ALTERNATIVES
EASIER   Small lifts, less repetitions
HARDER   Higher lifts (but don't overextend!), hands over head and finish with a set of 20 pulses in the highest position

---

PLUS (as often as possible!)
• Plank for >90 seconds
• >75 x pelvic tilt and head-lift combo (see page 90).

①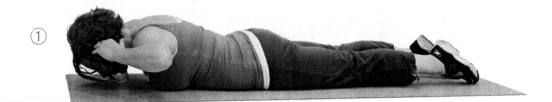

②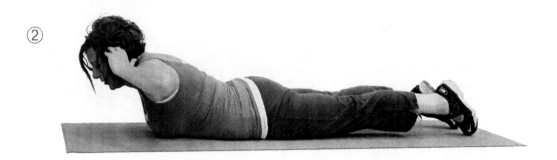

Pelvic floor exercises

The pelvic floor muscles are located between your legs and run from your pubic bone at the front to the base of your spine at the back. They give you control over your bladder and can be weakened by childbirth. But fear not! By doing some simple, regular exercises you will be able to strengthen them, whether you have already had your baby or not. Not only will these exercises help your bladder control, they may also increase the pleasure of having sex – so get started! If you have stitches during childbirth, these exercises will also help blood flow to the area to aid the healing process.

While you are doing your pelvic floor exercises, put your hands on your belly and buttocks to make sure you can't feel your belly, thighs or buttocks moving (unless the exercise specifies otherwise). Breathe normally and relax all other muscles. Don't squeeze your knees together or tense any other part of your body.

A quick way of finding the right muscles is by trying to stop the flow of urine when you're mid-flow – the correct movement is an upward and inward contraction. Don't make a habit of doing this on the toilet, though, as it is not good for you! You still need to do these exercises if you have a C-section as the weight of your baby will put pressure on your pelvic floor muscles. Try to do three of the exercises below (reps specified) five to seven times a week (and more often if you can). Make it easy for yourself – do them at work, on the bus or sitting watching TV. Exercises 6–11 are a bit harder and need a little more time, so if you're a busy lady just stick to the simple contractions – but make sure you do some!

1 Slow contractions

Slowly pull in your pelvic floor muscles. Hold for ten seconds and release. Repeat five times. This may be hard to start with, but try to build up to ten seconds.

2 Medium contractions

Pull in your pelvic floor muscles. Hold for two to three seconds (as tightly as possible) and release. Do this ten times. Repeat three times. This may be hard to start with, but try to build up to ten repetitions.

3 Fast contractions

Pull in your pelvic floor muscles. Hold for one second (as tightly as possible) and release. Do this ten times. This is like switching a light switch on and off. Repeat three times.

4 Progressive contractions

Pull in your pelvic floor muscles one-third of the way and hold. Pull them in another third and then hold. Pull them in all the way as tightly as you can and hold. Release using the same three steps. Repeat ten times.

5 Wave contractions

Pull in the muscles around your bottom, then all the way along to your front pelvic floors. Hold, then gradually release in a wave motion. Repeat ten times.

The following exercises may be hard to start with, but try to build up to ten repetitions:

6 Seated – knee push-down

With the soles of your feet together, apply slight pressure on top of your knees, pushing them to the floor, squeezing your pelvic floors. Push your knees back up against your hands. Hold for five seconds and release. Repeat ten times.

7 Seated – knee push-up

With the soles of your feet together, apply slight pressure from under your knees, pushing them up to the ceiling, squeezing your pelvic floors. Push your knees down against your hands. Hold for five seconds and release. Repeat ten times.

8 Standing – air cycles

Standing, using a chair for support, lift your leg to the side. Slowly circle your leg ten times one way, then ten times the other way, without putting it down and holding in your pelvic floors. Repeat twice on each side.

9 Standing – wall-squeezes

Stand with your shoulders and bottom against the wall. Pull your abdominals in so that your back is flat against the wall and pull your pelvic floors in. Hold for five seconds and release. Repeat ten times.

10 Pelvic tilt on all-fours – work your abs too!*

On all-fours with your back flat (this is essential), pull in your abdominals and hold. Then pull in your pelvic floor at the same time and hold. Release your pelvic floor muscles, then your abdominals. Repeat ten times.

11 Pelvic tilt lying on side – work your abs too!*

Lie on your side, with your body in a straight line and your lower leg bent back at 90 degrees behind you. Rest your head on your hand. Pull in your abdominals and hold, keeping your body straight. Your pelvis should tilt. Then pull in your pelvic floor at the same time and hold. Release your pelvic floor muscles, then your abdominals. Repeat ten times.

* As an alternative to 10 and 11, in Trimester 1 only (and after the birth) you can do a pelvic tilt on your back by pushing your lower back into the floor and hollowing the abdominals as you pull your abs and pelvic floors in. Your pelvis will tilt upwards as you pull the muscles in.

Common ailments

The path to becoming a new mum is not always a smooth one. Most women will have a low-risk pregnancy, but this does not mean that you will not experience discomforts, pains and niggles. Hopefully these won't stop you from exercising, but you may need to adapt your activity levels. Below are a few things you may experience and some advice. It's not all plain sailing ladies!

• •

These tips are taken from PregnancyFit 250, an app (coming in 2012) which you can download on your iphone. It gives you a daily tip, fact or snippet covering everything you need to know about exercise, diet, staying sane, lifestyle and your body during pregnancy. Add this to the 3-Plan to really build up your knowledge.

Sick as a pig Morning (or even all-day) sickness can be really unpleasant, but regular exercise and fresh air can help to ease it. Try to eat little and often; something plain such as crackers – ginger, peppermint and sniffing a lemon are also worth a try. Drink plenty of water and hope that it doesn't last long! See your doctor or midwife if it becomes severe.

Back way Many women get an achy lower back during pregnancy. Staying active can help prevent this. Also, try out a bump support and do regular back stretches (see page 22) to keep your muscles supple. If the pain becomes more severe in your back or pelvis then see your doctor or midwife.

Bless you! Its not pleasant when you are pregnant and have a cough or cold, even more so than

normal! Talk to a pharmacist about what medication is safe for you to take, drink plenty of water and eat well. Get plenty of rest and only do gentle exercise if you feel up to it.

Pile high Piles are common in pregnancy due to increased blood volume and relaxed blood vessels in your back bottom area. You can prevent them with good diet, hydration and exercise. If you do get them avoid scratching. They'll probably shrink when you have had your baby. The joys!

Skin deep Your skin undergoes all sorts of changes during pregnancy in terms of colour, itchiness, rashes, chaffing, stretch marks and veins – the glamour! Keep hydrated, moisturise and gently exfoliate regularly. Exercise and eating healthily will help minimise some of these symptoms, in part by contributing to a sensible, rather than excessive, weight gain.

Bleeding Don't panic if you get some bleeding during pregnancy. This is actually pretty common and there are lots of harmless reasons for it. However, if it is heavy or you are at all worried then get checked out. Seek medical attention immediately if the bleeding is a result of physical activity (this is highly unlikely).

Wrist action The increase in blood volume can cause wrists to swell and become painful, stiff, numb and tingly. This is called Carpal Tunnel Syndrome. If you suffer, avoid exercise that puts pressure on your wrists and heavy weights, use correct hand positions and see your doctor or midwife for advice.

Placenta previa This is a low-lying placenta, which can sit low early in pregnancy, then usually gradually moves around. However, if you are diagnosed with placenta previa after 26 weeks then you may have to hold off on the exercise. Your pregnancy will need to be carefully managed, so talk to your doctor or midwife.

Don't scratch! Thrush is common in pregnancy, but easily treatable and it won't affect your baby. You can use a pessary, with care (without the applicator), and apply cream, but don't take the oral capsules. Try to stay dry and cool down there! Chilled yoghurt applied directly is soothing, too. See your doctor or midwife for advice on treatment.

Bellyache It is not unusual to get tummy pains during pregnancy – there's a lot going on in there! They will come and go, but if the pain is severe or sustained or accompanied by bleeding or unusual discharge, then see your doctor or midwife.

Heartache As your bump grows you may suffer from painful heartburn and indigestion. Try to eat little and often and avoid spicy and rich foods. Drink water with meals and have a little walk afterwards.

Down under Cystitis and urinary tract infections are common in pregnancy due to the pressure of your growing uterus. Both can be very painful. Drink plenty of water, take warm baths to ease the discomfort and drink cranberry juice to help prevent future bouts. If you are suffering see your doctor or midwife.

Stitch in time A stitch in your side may become common as your bump grows. These can occur in your tummy or chest. To ease a stitch take a short rest from exercise to stretch (reach up and over), take deep breaths, drink water and start again slowly. Sometimes stitiches go; sometimes you just have to take a proper break.

Trial run Later on in your pregnancy you may notice Braxton Hicks (practice) contractions. This is when your womb tightens and your tum may go hard. Don't worry, they are completely normal (you are getting warmed up for the real thing!), but if they are painful or you have discharge or blood then see your doctor or midwife.

Cramp your style The dreaded cramp can be so painful – many swear words have been shouted due to night cramps! Exercise and stretching can prevent cramp, but if you do suffer then massage the area (usually your foot or leg), point and flex your foot, walk around or elevate it. Calcium in your diet may help, too. All part of the fun!

Herpes risk If you suffer from herpes then you will need to discuss this with your GP, especially if you get it for the first time while pregnant. This may also affect whether you can have a natural delivery as herpes can be passed on to your baby.

Wee-tastic Your growing bump will be putting extra pressure on your bladder, making you want to wee more. This is perfectly normal, but make sure, particularly if you are exercising, that you don't drink less. Stay well hydrated.

Lady lumps Cellulite affects most women, particularly as we get older. What can you do about it? Eat a good diet, exercise and drink lots of water – you should be doing this anyway! As for daily body-brushing – fab if you have the time, but the best advice is don't worry about a few bumpy bits!

Loch Ness Lochia is your womb lining coming out after you have had your baby (vaginally or by C-section). This bleeding varies from woman to woman but may last a few weeks. If it doesn't taper off or is an odd colour (i.e. very dark) see your doctor or midwife. Time to stock up on sanny pads!

Puffball Swollen ankles and feet are very common and caused by the extra blood in your system during pregnancy. To help put your feet up, get someone to rub them, drink plenty (yes!), keep up your exercise and stay away from your high heels!

Milky milky You may start to leak some pre-milk (colostrum) during Trimester 3. Now is the time to invest in some breast pads to put inside your bra, especially when you are exercising. BTW – the old wives' tale of cooled cabbage leaves in your bra to aid painful breasts later on really works!

Lightning strikes When your baby 'engages', the head drops into your pelvis, ready to come out. This can happen a few weeks or days before labour. Once this happens your bump may change shape, pressure eases on your diaphragm and you can breathe a bit more easily.

Liners You may experience a bit of wee wee leakage after you have had your baby, particularly when you exercise, sneeze or laugh. So start by wearing a panty liner (when the bleeding stops) and keep up those ever-important pelvic floors (I know – broken record!) If it affects your lifestyle, don't be embarrassed to see your doctor or midwife.

MORE SERIOUS STUFF...

High blood pressure? If you have high blood pressure then consult your GP before starting any exercise programme. It may be OK, depending on your circumstances, but you need to check as severe high blood pressure can cause serious problems in pregnancy if it is left unchecked.

Diabetes Exercise lowers your risk of gestational diabetes, which is caused by a rise in insulin during pregnancy. Another big plus! However, if you find yourself weeing all the time and are always thirsty, it is best to talk to your doctor or midwife just to be sure.

Pre-eclampsia You'll need to have regular blood pressure checks as pre-eclampsia can develop after 20 weeks. This is severe high blood pressure (and protein in your wee) and can cause complications for you and your baby if it is not managed carefully.

Ouch! Some women suffer from very severe pelvic pain as their ligaments relax and the pelvis enlarges. This may be Symphysis Pubis Dysfunction (SFD). and it can also be felt in the back. It can be agonising and needs medical attention. You will not be able to do regular exercise with SPD.

What happens now?

Now nine months have passed since you had your baby and I hope you have enjoyed the 3-Plan and are looking and feeling fantastic! The aim of this plan is not to get you healthy for a month or a year, but to get you into the exercise habit for the rest of your life.

Now you have got to the end, you could start from the beginning and work through the 3-Plan again, pushing yourself even harder than before. You can mix and match any of the exercises (there are over 75 to choose from!) to put together your own plan – just don't choose all the easy ones! Or you could try a completely new type of exercise.

The underlying principle of this plan is to make healthy, active choices whenever you can and to fit exercise in around your lifestyle. If that becomes your mantra – you are set for life. Whatever you do, please keep it up; if you don't use it, you lose it!

And remember to pick up the 3-Plan again if you decide to add to your family in future years!

Please write to me with any comments or feedback: email: info@bump2mumfitness.com – I would love you hear from you.

Web: www.bump2mumfitness.com
Facebook: www.facebook.com/bump2mumfitness
Twitter: bump2mumfit
Blog: bump2mumfitness.blogspot.com

EXERCISE JOURNAL TEMPLATES

Print one of these off for each week you are following the 3-Plan and use it to motivate yourself! Try and meet your goals each week. One is provided to get you started; you can print off more of these templates at www.bump2mumfitness.com.

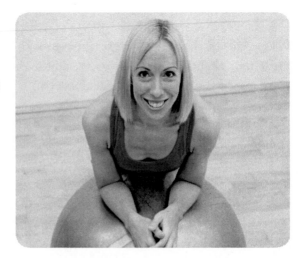

3-PLAN EXERCISE JOURNAL TEMPLATE

		Tick when done	Actual time spent/details
Resistance session 1	Aim – programme 30-40 minutes		
Resistance session 2	Aim – programme 30-40 minutes		
Resistance session 3	Aim – programme 30-40 minutes		
Resistance session extra (optional)	Aim – programme 30-40 minutes		
	Total number and time spent this week =	i.e. 3 sessions	i.e. 1 and a half hrs
	Goal =	**3-4 sessions**	**1 and half hrs– 2 hrs and 40 mins**

CARDIO :

		Tick when done	Actual time spent/details
Cardio session 1 (Moderate – high)	Aim – programme 30-60 minutes		
Cardio session 2 (Moderate – high)	Aim – programme 30-60 minutes		
Cardio session 3 (Moderate – high)	Aim – programme 30-60 minutes		
Cardio session 4 extra (optional)	Aim – programme 30-60 minutes		
Cardio session 5 extra (optional)	Aim – programme 30-60 minutes		
	Total number and time spent this week =	i.e. 3 sessions	i.e. 1 and a half hrs
	Goal =	**3-6 sessions**	**1 and half hrs– 5 hours**

Weekly total (3-Plan + cardio = _____(Goal 3 hours–7 hours 20 min)

EXTRAS

Pelvic floor exercises – aim for daily (tick under number when done):

1	2	3	4	5	6	7

Extra – bottom squeezes - aim for daily (tick under number when done):

1	2	3	4	5	6	7

Extra – Ab squeezes - aim for daily (tick under number when done):

1	2	3	4	5	6	7

3-PLAN EXERCISE JOURNAL TEMPLATE

		Tick when done	Actual time spent/details
Resistance session 1	Aim – programme 30-40 minutes		
Resistance session 2	Aim – programme 30-40 minutes		
Resistance session 3	Aim – programme 30-40 minutes		
Resistance session extra (optional)	Aim – programme 30-40 minutes		
	Total number and time spent this week =	i.e. 3 sessions	i.e. 1 and a half hrs
	Goal =	**3-4 sessions**	**1 and half hrs– 2 hrs and 40 mins**

CARDIO :

		Tick when done	Actual time spent/details
Cardio session 1 (Moderate – high)	Aim – programme 30-60 minutes		
Cardio session 2 (Moderate – high)	Aim – programme 30-60 minutes		
Cardio session 3 (Moderate – high)	Aim – programme 30-60 minutes		
Cardio session 4 extra (optional)	Aim – programme 30-60 minutes		
Cardio session 5 extra (optional)	Aim – programme 30-60 minutes		
	Total number and time spent this week =	i.e. 3 sessions	i.e. 1 and a half hrs
	Goal =	**3-6 sessions**	**1 and half hrs– 5 hours**

Weekly total (3-Plan + cardio = _____(Goal 3 hours–7 hours 20 min)

EXTRAS

Pelvic floor exercises – aim for daily (tick under number when done):

1	2	3	4	5	6	7

Extra – bottom squeezes - aim for daily (tick under number when done):

1	2	3	4	5	6	7

Extra – Ab squeezes - aim for daily (tick under number when done):

1	2	3	4	5	6	7

THE MODELS HAVE THEIR SAY

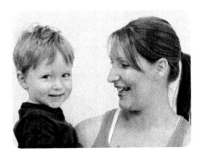

"I'll definitely be using the book, especially once I've had the baby, as I am getting married abroad next year and have a beautiful wedding dress to fit into!" Carli

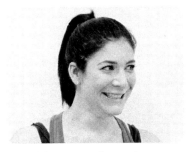

"It's odd to see my figure change shape so dramatically but I'm enjoying every minute of it!"
Wendy

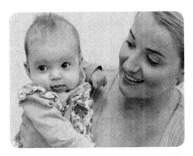

"Being a mum to my gorgeous girl, Scarlett, is the most rewarding experience of my life. Working out to get my body back is easier than I thought and I can fit it in around looking after her." Steph

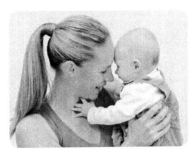

"The whole experience of motherhood for me has been amazing, from pregnancy to now – and even the birth! I can't quite believe I can say that. She really has fitted beautifully into our lives and I have been able to keep active. I'm a new mum, learning every day, and cherishing each moment." Jo

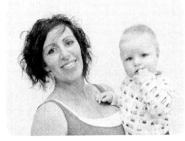

"I am married with three children ages 19, 13 and 8 months. Most of my general exercise is walking and running around after children! I try to eat a balanced healthy diet but do have the odd glass of red wine."
Simone

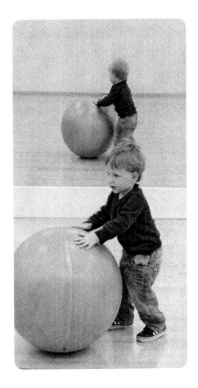

RESOURCES

Helplines and websites for further information and advice about pregnancy and post-natal issues:

National Breastfeeding helpline, 0300 100 0210 (www.nationalbreastfeedinghelpline.org.uk)

National Childbirth Trust (NCT), 0300 330 0770 (www.nct.org.uk)

NHS pregnancy smoking helpline, Weekdays 9–8pm, Weekends 11–5pm, 0800 0224 332 (www.smokefree.nhs.uk)

Antenatal Results and Choices, Weekdays 10am–5.30pm, 0207 631 0285 (www.arc-uk.org)

Action on Pre-eclampsia, 01386 761848 (www.apec.org.uk)

Twins & Multiple Births Assoc. (Twinline), 0800 138 0509 (www.tamba.org.uk)

Association for Postnatal Illness, Mon–Fri 10–2 pm, 0207 386 0868 (www.apni.org)

Cry-sis (crying baby), 9am-10pm, 0845 122 8669 (www.cry-sis.org.uk)

Rise (domestic abuse), 01273 622 822 (www.riseuk.org.uk)

Association of Breastfeeding Mothers, 08444 122 949, (abm.me.uk)

La Leche League, 0845 120 2918 (www.laleche.org.uk)

Breastfeeding Network, 0300 100 0210 (www.breastfeedingnetwork.org.uk)

Hypnobirthing – to read more and find a class in your area (www.hypnobirthing.co.uk)

Netmums – chat, advice, resources, information and more (www.netmums.com)

Independent Midwives – read more about independent midwives in the UK (www. independentmidwives.org.uk)

National Institute for Health and Clinical Excellence (NICE) – for up to date clinical guidance (www.nice.org.uk)

Royal College of Obstetricians and Gynaecologists (RCOG) (www.rcog.org.uk)

Royal College of Midwives (www.rcm.org.uk)

Nursing and Midwifery Council (www.nmc-uk.org)

ACKNOWLEDGEMENTS

I would very much like to thank…..

My gorgeous models and their bumps and babies who helped out just for the fun of it: Carli Adamski, Wendy Butler, Jo Emery, Steph Lyndon-James and Simone Thorn.

Samantha Shearman, local portrait photographer for the fab photos.
(http://sites.google.com/site/angeleyesimages/)

Amy from Beauty Box in Shoreham-by-sea for the stunning make-up.
(www.thebeautyboxshoreham.com)

Impulse Leisure for letting us use the studio at Southwick for our photoshoot.
(www.impulseleisure.co.uk)

And most importantly:
Peggy Sadler and Jo Godfrey Wood at Bookworx for producing my book and turning my words and ideas into a thing of beauty.
(www.bookworx.biz)

Lightning Source UK Ltd.
Milton Keynes UK
UKOW021934030912

198434UK00008B/102/P